Harold G. Koenig, MD, MHSc

# Is Religion Good f...
## The Effects o...
## on Physical and N...

*Pre-publication*
*REVIEWS,*
*COMMENTARIES,*
*EVALUATIONS . . .*

"*Is Religion Good for Your Health?* is a fascinating study. Pastors, people in churches, and anyone concerned with religion or health (or both) will be fascinated by Dr. Koenig's work. After nearly a century of some suspicion about the negative relationship between religion and good mental health, Dr. Koenig suggests that the relationship between these two concerns may be more beneficial than we had thought. This book will be talked about for a long time."

**William H. Willimon**
*Dean of the Chapel and Professor of Christian Ministry,*
*Duke University Chapel,*
*Durham, NC*

"Finally, a systematic review of the effects of healthy religion on the well-being of people. Koenig leads the reader through one piece of research after another that demonstrates the positive health possibilities and actualities of religious experience. Upbeat, forward-looking, and constructive, *Is Religion Good for Your Health?* abandons clichés and unwarranted personal biases and lets the research do the talking. This is a book designed for earnest personal reflection and use as a basis to foster the wholistic care of people."

**Bruce M. Hartung, PhD**
*Director, Health Ministries,*
*Lutheran Church,*
*Missouri Synod,*
*Kirkwood, MO*

"**M**any health professionals trivialize the importance of religion in the lives and health of Americans and some actually characterize it as a negative and neurotic influence on the mental health of individuals. These views are usually based on stereotypes or limited clinical experiences. In *Is Religion Good for Your Health?*, family physician, psychiatrist, and researcher Dr. Harold Koenig presents a compelling, balanced overview of the scientific research examining the relationship between religion and health (much of which has been conducted by Dr. Koenig or his colleagues at Duke University). He concludes that a wide array of studies using different methodologies have demonstrated rather strongly that religious belief and practice have positive effects on both mental and physical health.

Given the aging of the baby boomer cohort and health-care funding pressures, it is essential that creative energy be given to developing innovative and cost-effective strategies for health education, information and referral, and the delivery of health care. In a thought-provoking final chapter, Koenig discusses the implications of the findings of research on the health-religion connection for health professionals, clergy, public policy-makers, medical researchers, and laypersons. He suggests that religious beliefs and practices may provide a rich resource for individuals to draw on to enhance both mental and physical health.

This is an important book that moves beyond stereotypes of religion and its effects on health by using the window of science to inform and enlighten the reader. Concise and readable, it contains a wealth of helpful charts and figures to visually depict the information contained in the text. The book is recommended for busy professionals and laypersons alike."

**Brian F. Hofland, PhD**
*Senior Vice President,*
*The Retirement Research Foundation,*
*Chicago, IL*

The Haworth Pastoral Press
An Imprint of The Haworth Press, Inc.

# Is Religion Good for Your Health?
## *The Effects of Religion on Physical and Mental Health*

# HAWORTH Religion and Mental Health
## Harold G. Koenig, MD
### Senior Editor

*A Gospel for the Mature Years: Finding Fulfillment by Knowing and Using Your Gifts* by Harold Koenig, Tracy Lamar, and Betty Lamar

*Is Religion Good for Your Health? The Effects of Religion on Physical and Mental Health* by Harold Koenig

Additional Titles of Related Interest:

*Growing Up: Pastoral Nurture for the Later Years* by Thomas B. Robb

*Religion and the Family: When God Helps* by Laurel Arthur Burton

*Victims of Dementia: Services, Support, and Care* by Wm. Michael Clemmer

*Horrific Traumata: A Pastoral Response to the Post-Traumatic Stress Disorder* by N. Duncan Sinclair

*Aging and God: Spiritual Pathways to Mental Health in Midlife and Later Years* by Harold G. Koenig

*Counseling for Spiritually Empowered Wholeness: A Hope-Centered Approach* by Howard Clinebell

*Shame: A Faith Perspective* by Robert H. Albers

*Dealing with Depression: Five Pastoral Interventions* by Richard Dayringer

*Righteous Religion: Unmasking the Illusions of Fundamentalism and Authoritarian Catholicism* by Kathleen Y. Ritter and Craig W. O'Neill

*Theological Context for Pastoral Caregiving: Word in Deed* by Howard Stone

*Pastoral Care in Pregnancy Loss: A Ministry Long Needed* by Thomas Moe

*The Soul in Distress: What Every Pastoral Counselor Should Know About Emotional and Mental Illness* by Richard Roukema

# Is Religion Good for Your Health?
## *The Effects of Religion on Physical and Mental Health*

Harold G. Koenig, MD, MHSc

The Haworth Pastoral Press
An Imprint of The Haworth Press, Inc.
New York • London

Published by

The Haworth Pastoral Press, an imprint of The Haworth Press, Inc., 10 Alice Street, Binghamton, NY 13904-1580

**Library of Congress Cataloging-in-Publication Data**

Koenig, Harold George.
    Is religion good for your health? : the effects of religion on physical and mental health / Harold G. Koenig.
       p.  cm.
    Includes bibliographical references and index.
    ISBN 0-7890-0229-9 (pbk. : alk. paper).         0-7890-0166-7
    1. Health–Religious aspects. 2. Mental health–Religious aspects. 3. United States–Statistics, Medical. 4. United States–Statistics, Vital. 5. United States–Religion–1960. I. Title.
BL65.M4K64 1997
200′.1′3–dc21

                                      96-48053
                                        CIP

To Charmin, my lovely wife;
Jordan, my strong and handsome son;
and Rebekah, my precious little girl.

# ABOUT THE AUTHOR

**Harold G. Koenig, MD, MHSc,** completed his undergraduate education at Stanford University, his medical school training at the University of California at San Francisco, and his geriatric medicine, psychiatry, and biostatistics training at Duke University Medical Center. He is currently on the faculty at Duke University as an Associate Professor of Psychiatry and an Assistant Professor of Internal Medicine, and is director of the *Program on Religion, Aging, and Health*. Dr. Koenig has published extensively in the fields of mental health, geriatrics, and religion, with over 100 scientific articles, 22 book chapters, and seven books. His research on religion and health has been featured on National Public Radio, *ABC World News Tonight*, *NBC Evening News*, *CBS Evening News* and *CBS Morning News*, Ivanhoe Broadcast News, and in journals and newspapers such as *Arthritis Today*, *The Daily Telegraph* (London*)*, *The Guardian* (Europe), and other local, national, and international programs and periodicals. In 1995, he was one of the conveners of a conference sponsored by the National Institute on Aging on the topic of "Religion, Aging, and Health," and in 1996 he organized a symposium on religion and health at the American Association for the Advancement of Science, the largest science organization in the world. He is the recipient of a five-year Mental Health Academic Award from the National Institute of Mental Health to study depression in older persons with medical illness. As well, he has received grants from the Retirement Research Foundation and the Sir John Templeton Foundation to study the relationship between religion and health.

# CONTENTS

**Foreword**                                                ix
            *David O. Moberg*

**Introduction**                                             1

**Chapter 1: Mrs. Bernard's Story**                          5

**Chapter 2: Societal Trends in the Twentieth
     and Twenty-First Centuries**                            9

Demographic Trends                                          10
Health Trends                                               11
Family Trends                                               15
Economic Trends                                             17
Community Resources                                         19
Summary                                                     19

**Chapter 3: Negative Effects of Religion on Health**       23

Sigmund Freud                                               23
Albert Ellis                                                25
Wendell Watters                                             26
Other Mental Health Professionals                           27
Primary Care Physicians                                     28
Summary                                                     30

**Chapter 4: Are Americans Becoming Less Religious?**       33

Religious Beliefs                                           33
Importance of Religion                                      36
Influence of Religion on Life                               36
Religious Affiliation                                       37
Church Membership                                           38
Church Attendance                                           38
Religious Television                                        43

Prayer................................................................43
Bible Reading....................................................44
Religion and Aging.............................................44
Summary...........................................................46

**Chapter 5: Religion and Mental Health**........**49**

Religious Coping................................................50
Well-Being and Life Satisfaction.........................53
Depression and Suicide.......................................55
Anxiety.............................................................63
Alcohol and Drug Abuse......................................63
Treatment Studies..............................................66
Possible Mechanisms of Effect............................67
Summary...........................................................71

**Chapter 6: Religion and Physical Health**.......**77**

Direct and Indirect Influences.............................78
Diseases of the Blood Vessels and Heart...............82
Cancer.............................................................90
All-Cause Mortality...........................................92
Summary...........................................................93

**Chapter 7: Conclusions and Reanalysis**........**101**

Effects on Mental Health....................................101
Effects on Physical Health..................................102
Pathological Aspects of Religion Reanalyzed.........104
Summary...........................................................111

**Chapter 8: Implications**...............................**119**

Health Professionals..........................................119
Religious Professionals.......................................122
Public Policymakers...........................................124
Medical Researchers..........................................125
Laypersons.......................................................126
Summary...........................................................127

**General Reviews of the Research Literature**....**129**

**Index**..........................................................**131**

# Foreword

The myth of a Fountain of Youth has enticed many people through the centuries. Juan Ponce de León, Hernando de Soto, and Pánfilo de Narváez are among the sixteenth-century Spanish explorers who were motivated, at least in part, by that legend to search for the fountain in the New World of America that is now part of the United States. The natives of Central America believed as well that a mystical spring somewhere to their north gave water that would cure human ills and restore youth to those who drank it.

We still seek the Fountain of Youth—no longer in the naive belief that it is an actual spring of waters that miraculously brings healing and youth, but rather in the sophisticated modern faith that medical, pharmaceutical, and genetic scientific research will eventually uncover all mysteries of human disability, illness, and aging, thus enabling us to live longer and happier lives or perhaps even to find an earthly immortality for our grandchildren, if not for ourselves.

In this search, many areas of the complex interdisciplinary field known as gerontology, the science of aging, have received extensive attention, so much so that one could quite correctly say that it has become a flourishing new science. At the same time, the study of religion and aging has languished and lagged behind. Only recently has religious gerontology begun to attain a position of respect within the health-related professions. This has occurred partly as a result of societal trends. It also is a result of significant research done by many scholars and scientists, among whom David B. Larson, Jeffrey S. Levin, and Harold G. Koenig, the author of this book, are especially prominent. They have firmly established that religion, especially Christianity (which is the most studied), is an important ingredient in the life-enhancing "waters" of a modern "fountain of youth."

In this book, Koenig summarizes much of what has been discovered through his own and others' research related to the question of whether religion is, as claimed by many of its adherents, a "balm of Gilead" or, as claimed by influential nonbelievers, a "deadly doctrine" that is a curse upon humanity. From the perspective of science, this is a difficult question to answer because research focused on relationships between religion and health has long been suspected of bearing an incurable bias. The tendency of religiously devout people and clergy, on the one hand, and of atheists and agnostics on the other, usually has been to indulge in "card stacking"–accumulating every shred of evidence that supports their preconceived conclusions while ignoring all evidence that contradicts it. Even when done with the best of motives, this approach not only violates the principles of the search for verified knowledge, known collectively as "the scientific method," but it also constitutes the despicable sin of "bearing false witness" whenever the findings are deceitfully presented as if they constitute the whole story.

Honesty and integrity demand that evidence be sought on both or all sides of any issue, which is what Dr. Koenig has done in this book. He examines and summarizes the research findings both for and against the proposition that religion is good for one's health, and he does so with ample documentation of published sources so that readers can locate and examine the details of the original studies upon which his generalizations are based.

The focus of this book is on physical and mental health as conventionally defined in relation to religion. Almost no attention is given to the "softer" social and behavioral science research on the relationship of religion to such health-related subjects as peace of mind, happiness, morale, quality of life, and life satisfaction, although the general direction of findings on those subjects is similar. As early as 1951, there were already several such studies. My research on religion and personal adjustment to old age revealed that higher levels of religious beliefs and activities, not limited to religious affiliation or church membership, were significantly associated with higher levels of personal adjustment to old age, and vice versa. Subsequent research has consistently revealed similar relationships. The self-reports and subjective data from survey research in the social and behavioral sciences thus lend credence to findings from the more objective studies on physical and mental health that are summarized in this book.

Here, then, is strong, tangible, scientific evidence to answer the question, "Is religion good for your health?" It is not based simply on testimonials and one-sided case studies of devout people who believe that "Prayer changes things" (technically meaning that "God changes things when believers pray"). Neither is it founded on the reductionistic tendency of those scientists and scholars who discount the wholesome influence of religion completely, reinterpreting findings of its effects as due to little or nothing more than wishful thinking, psychosomatic healing, stereotyped answers in interviews or survey questions, or such phenomena as a person's social integration into a religious group or the self-healing mechanisms of the human body and mind.

Because Christianity is the dominant religion in the United States, most of the research on "religion and health" to date actually pertains to "Christianity and health." In summarizing it, Dr. Koenig wisely narrows most of the work reported here to religious commitment, beliefs, and practices, omitting numerous studies that define the religion variable as merely self-identification with a religious ideology, sect, or denomination, or an alleged affiliation with a broad category such as "Protestant, Catholic, Jew, Other, or

None." The findings of studies based on those loose operational definitions of "religion" seldom contradict those reported here, but the relationships with measures of health included in them are often more tenuous and much weaker, largely because they include so many people whose religion consists mainly of a family heritage or "membership" extrinsically imposed upon them by parents, ethnic identity, or the need for respectability in their profession or community, in contrast to an intrinsic personal choice based on a sincere faith commitment.

As a medical doctor and psychiatrist, Dr. Koenig has a strong base of clinical experience related to this subject. As a researcher skilled in survey methodology and epidemiological investigation, he is extraordinarily capable of evaluating the strengths and weaknesses of the research done by others. As a therapist, he empathizes with the reservations and fears of patients who yearn for healing. As a teacher, he understands the challenges brought by skeptical students and faculty colleagues to any broad generalization about cause-and-effect relationships. As the author of several related survey books, he has an exceptional grasp of current knowledge of this subject. Only those who refuse to allow factual research findings to speak for themselves will dislike this fascinating summary of research findings related to religion and health.

Here, then, is a compendium of the solidly established evidence for both the "Yes" and the "No" answers to the question of whether religion influences health in a positive way. It is couched in language that any reader of English can understand. It emphasizes tangible scientific data, not mere dogma, myth, and folklore, and is accompanied by specific references to the many sources that together help to provide the answers. Although the evidence seems to pile up heavily in one direction, Dr. Koenig carefully qualifies his conclusions, knowing that scientific findings seldom, if ever, are absolute and final.

More research is still needed on this fascinating subject. This summary of findings-to-date suggests dozens of topics for such investigations and provides many background leads to future studies with the help of pertinent previous investigations.

Despite Dr. Koenig's compelling conclusions, you personally may not find the answer to the question of whether religion is good for your own health. Pastors, chaplains, counselors, other therapists, and friends can also help you to find your personal answer. They can guide your probe of issues related to such questions as your personal definition or interpretation of what is "good," what you include under the concept of "health," your concept of "religion" and which specific manifestation of it (congregation, parish, fellowship group, etc.) is under consideration, and many other particular circumstances in your own life. You and they will surely find much help here.

Certainly a religion used pathologically will almost inevitably have some negative effects on your physical and mental health, even if the predominant influence of most American religion tends to be in the opposite positive direction. In addition, it is not yet clear whether "becoming religious" only for the sake of restoring or improving one's health will by itself contribute to the desired result.

The typical focus of attention in personal conversations about religion, as well as in discussions about it in many college classrooms, the press, and the other mass media, tends to be on whatever is unusual or spectacular. Yet the non-newsworthy religion that is typical, customary, and normally experienced and expected by the vast majority of people, which is the basis of most studies reported here, undoubtedly has far greater effects on the personal lives of most people and is more influential in society.

Is religion an ingredient of the elixir of the Fountain of Youth? Read on to discover its significant effects on health that are firmly documented by systematic research!

*David O. Moberg, PhD*
*Sociology Professor Emeritus,*
*Marquette University*

# Introduction

Science without religion is lame, religion without science is blind.

—Albert Einstein
(*Science, Philosophy and Religion*, 1941)

This book explores a question that has been debated for centuries: "Is religion good for your health?" The clergy preach eloquently about the comfort and consolation that religious faith brings to the devout. Some health professionals, on the contrary, argue that such faith is either irrelevant or damaging to health. As a family physician and later as a psychiatrist, I grappled with this question as well. Over the past 20 years, I have listened to many patients talk about their health, their sufferings, and their faith. What role might religion be playing in these patients' health or illnesses, I wondered.

While the debate over religion's positive or negative influences on health has raged for hundreds, perhaps thousands of years, until the past 50 years there has been no substantial effort to objectively and systematically examine the question. Considerable research, much of which occurred at Duke University during the past decade, has now carefully examined the relationship between religion and health. What have researchers found? In this book, I will review some of this research and discuss the findings. The answer to the question, "Is religion good for your health?" is relevant for health professionals and for pastoral counselors, because it touches on the very heart of what these professions are about.

In the first chapter, I briefly tell a story about my experience with Mrs. Bernard that recounts how I first became interested in this area over ten years ago. In the second chapter, I examine trends in society over the past century and projections of these trends into the next century: aging of the American population, changes in physical and mental health, changes in attitudes and values, changes in family structure, and changes in the financing of health care. In the third chapter, I explore concerns about religion's negative effects on health as articulated by Sigmund Freud, Albert Ellis, Wendell Watters, and other health experts, who have argued that religion and health are actually inimical to each other. In the fourth chapter, I look at how important religion is to Americans and examine to what extent its influence in secular America is waning.

The fifth and sixth chapters are the heart of this book. Here I present and discuss the results of recent research that first examined the relationship between religion and mental health, and then the relationship between religion and physical health. In Chapter 7, I succinctly review the major research findings and discuss what we can conclude from these findings. Also in this chapter, I review and reanalyze the pathological aspects of religion, using an approach enlightened by recent research in order to achieve a deeper and more balanced understanding of the effects of religion on psychopathology and vice versa. In the final chapter, I examine the implications of this research for health professionals (physicians, nurses, and social workers), religious professionals (community clergy, chaplains, and pastoral counselors), public policy experts, medical researchers, and laypersons.

This book is intended for health professionals, religious professionals, social and behavioral scientists, public policy experts, medical researchers, and students in any of these fields, who are looking for a relatively concise review of the research examining the religion/health relationship and are seeking to understand the importance and implications of this research. While intended primarily for an academic audience, this volume will also interest the general reader. Persons born prior to 1946 and between 1946 and 1965 (baby boomers) will find the information contained here especially enlightening, if not a bit disturbing, since it addresses changes presently occurring in society that will directly affect their lives and the lives of their children and grandchildren.

The book contains many figures and graphs that visually depict trends over time and relationships between religion and health outcomes. These will give the reader a better sense of the magnitude of the relationships and will be useful for teaching purposes. There is also an extensive reference list that readers may consult if they wish to verify results themselves. Following the citations from the text, the section on general reviews of the religion/health literature will lead the reader to many research studies not reviewed here. Finally, at the end of the book there is a detailed subject index that will allow quick and easy access to topics of special interest.

# Chapter 1

# Mrs. Bernard's Story

I walked into Mrs. Bernard's room and introduced myself. I was on morning rounds at the hospital, and had just learned that this patient, admitted with a hip fracture four weeks ago, would be discharged later in the day. I was scheduled to see her next week, so I decided to stop by and check on her before she went home. Mrs. Bernard had endured a complicated and stormy hospital stay over the past month. When referring the case to me, her surgeon told me that Mrs. Bernard had lost her only son in a tragic car accident six months previously. Only five weeks ago her husband had died suddenly from a stroke, leaving her alone in a large metropolitan city. A week after that, while attending his funeral, she slipped on the ice and fractured her hip. While recovering from the hip fracture, she developed a bad infection in her lungs, which required a prolonged stay in the hospital. The surgeon, concerned about how she was handling all this, suggested I see her before she was discharged.

When I walked into Mrs. Bernard's room, I found her reading her Bible. She looked up and smiled. In a friendly voice she said, "Hello. Dr. Jones said you'd be by today. Come sit down." I pulled up a chair, feeling a bit more relaxed myself after hearing the friendly tone in her greeting. She set the Bible down next to her and said, "What can I do for you doctor?" I explained that I would be seeing her in my clinic the following week and relayed some of the concerns her surgeon had about how she was handling the stress in her life. Mrs. Bernard admitted to being sad over the loss of her son and husband, but said she was thankful she still had a loving and devoted daughter in Tennessee and was planning to move closer to her after she completed rehabilitation for her hip fracture. At first I thought she was in denial, a mechanism by which the mind pushes stressful experiences out of consciousness. After talking with her for about ten minutes, however, I realized she was thinking quite rationally and seemed to be handling the stress quite well, much better than most persons in her situation.

I asked curiously, "Mrs. Bernard, all things considered, you seem to be handling things fairly well despite these painful losses in your life. Most people would be pretty upset about all this. But you seem calm and accepting. What is your secret? What enables you to cope the way you do?" She was silent for a moment. She picked up her Bible. A smile came across her face. "This is what helps me," she said. "Whenever I get to feeling sad or blue, I pick up my Bible and begin reading it, and somehow this calms me." I encouraged her to elaborate, saying, "So your religion has been a help to you?" "Oh, yes," she responded. "It's the most important thing that's kept me going. When I wake up at night and feel alone or afraid, I read my Bible or talk to God. He's always there, even when my family and friends are not."

Mrs. Bernard was like hundreds of other patients I came across who used religion as a source of comfort when facing severe medical illness or personal crisis. In my early years as a family physician, I would frequently come across patients in the hospital who were praying, saying the rosary, reading their Bible, or watching religious programs on television. I became curious about these behaviors and began asking patients why they were doing this. Invariably, they told me that these religious activities helped them to better deal with their illness.

This was back in the early 1980s. To find out more about the subject, I searched medical literature hoping to discover something about the effect of religious behaviors on health. I found almost nothing in the standard medical journals, and what I did find talked about the harmful or neurotic effects of religion. For this reason, I decided to conduct some research of my own. Religion's effects on health, I thought, should be easiest to study among persons experiencing severe personal crisis–those who were physically ill, hospitalized with life-threatening illness, or in some other difficult life situation. Such circumstances seriously test a person's coping resources. Their use of religion (if any) would provide important clues about whether it did or did not facilitate coping, adaptation, and healing. It would also expose whether religion signified weakness or psychological instability, or if it exerted any adverse effects on mental health. Finally, the positive or negative effects of religion on physical health would be easiest to see in persons who were most vulnerable–the sick, the frail, the elderly.

For almost 15 years now, our research group has been studying how religious beliefs and activities influence health. This book contains the results of over ten major research studies conducted at Duke University on this topic and briefly summarizes the findings of other investigators working in different areas of the United States who have attempted to answer the intriguing and controversial question, "Is religion good for your health?"

What do I mean by the word "religion"? Religion as used here primarily involves traditional Judeo-Christian beliefs and practices. These include depth of belief in and commitment to God; frequency of prayer, scripture reading, church or synagogue attendance; and the use of these beliefs and practices when coping with stress. I deal very little with the broader issue of spirituality or with nontraditional New Age spiritual beliefs or practices, although these are briefly addressed in Chapter 5.

Read on to discover the answer to the question of religion's influence on health that science is helping to provide.

# Chapter 2

# Societal Trends in the Twentieth and Twenty-First Centuries

Before discussing the relationship between religion and health, let us examine demographic, health, family, and economic changes that have been rapidly occurring in the United States and throughout the world during the past century. This will provide a background for religion's influence on health and society. Many of these changes have been driven by advances in science and technology. Progress in telecommunications allows us to speak with relatives and friends in distant countries at any time of the day or night, watch every detail of a war on the other side of the globe, make purchases or business transactions on the Internet, all from the comfort and safety of home.

While technological improvements have markedly enhanced our lifestyles, they have not been achieved without a price. In order to afford these and other luxuries which have become the norm in American society, most families require both parents to work outside the home. A single working parent is often no longer able to earn enough money to afford a three bedroom home, health and life insurance, a newer model car, cable TV, the newest computer and accessories, and other aspects of the modern lifestyle. There is little time left in this quick-paced world to communicate intimately with our spouses, listen to the growing pains of our children, care for our elderly parents, or help or even get to know our neighbors. These trends, together with a shift in the age distribution of our population and advances in medicine and health care, are having increasingly unsettling consequences.

## DEMOGRAPHIC TRENDS

The post-World War II baby boom resulted in the birth of 74 million persons between 1945 and 1965. Advances in health care have greatly reduced infant and childhood mortality at one end of the life spectrum,[1] and prolonged life through treatments of cancer, heart disease, and other chronic illnesses, at the other end.[2] This, together with a declining birth rate, has caused the aging of our population.[3] In 1900, there were only about 3 million persons age 65 or older in the United States, comprising about 4 percent of the total population; in 1990, the figure was 12.5 percent; and by the year 2030, 20 percent of Americans will be age 65 or over[4] (see Figure 2.1). In fact, a baby girl born today in the United States can expect to live into her nineties and a baby boy into his eighties.

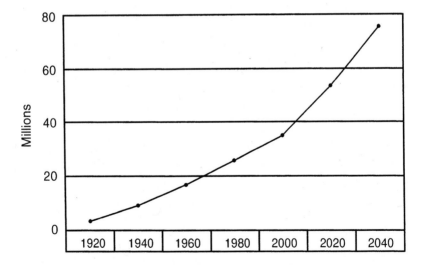

FIGURE 2.1. Population 65 Years or Older, 1920-2040

Source: Schick and Schick (1994). *Statistical Handbook on Aging Americans* (series #5). New York: Oryx Press.

## HEALTH TRENDS

If people were living longer, healthier, and happier lives, with fewer physical health problems and less disabilities, then there would be no need for anything but optimism and hope for the future. However, there is increasing evidence that this is not what is happening. Yes, people are living longer, but often with a chronic illness that is disabling and very expensive to treat. Kunkel and Applebaum,[5] based on information from two national data sets, projected that while there were only about 2 million severely disabled persons age 65 or over in the United States in 1980, the figure would increase almost sixfold by the year 2040 (see Figure 2.2). These figures do not include persons with milder forms of long-term disability, a number that may reach almost 23 million. Likewise, whereas only about 2 to 4 million

FIGURE 2.2. Projected Number of Severely Disabled Persons Over Age 65

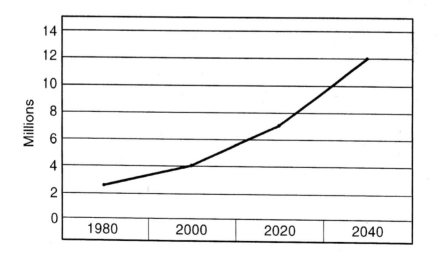

Source: Kunkel and Applebaum (1992). *Journal of Gerontology* 47: S253-S260.

persons today experience Alzheimer's disease, this figure could rise to as high as 14 million in the next 50 years[6] (see Figure 2.3). Who is going to care for this rapidly expanding chronically ill, disabled elderly population in the years ahead?

The situation worsens when we consider the increasing mental health needs of our population, particularly those of younger and middle-aged persons (baby boomers). The current generation of older adults in the United States has lived through hard economic times and one or two world wars. It has often grappled with disabling physical health problems or other losses associated with aging. Despite this, however, older adults experience relatively low rates of depression, alcohol abuse, drug abuse, and other mental health problems. In 1980, only 7 out of 1000 per-

FIGURE 2.3. Number of Cases of Alzheimer's Disease, 1960-2050

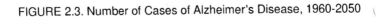

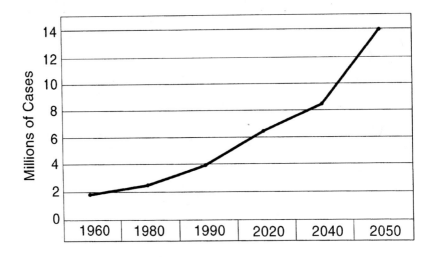

Based on 10 percent of the population over age 65 and 47 percent of those over age 85 with Alzheimer's Disease.

Source: Evans et al. (1989). *Journal of the American Medical Association* 262:2551-2556.

sons age 65 or over experienced a serious problem with depression, compared with 25 out of 1000 persons between ages 18 and 45 years (over three times as many).[7] In 1980, alcohol and drug abuse were present in fewer than 10 out of 1000 persons age 65 or over, compared with 65 out of 1000 persons ages 18 to 45 (six times more common). If one multiplies the 1980 rates of depression and alcohol/drug abuse in baby boomers by the number of persons in this population group, and projects the resulting figures into the future about 40 years, it is evident that the number of older persons with mental health problems will increase dramatically (see Figure 2.4).

Unfortunately, these calculations probably *underestimate* the problem looming ahead. The above figures fail to account for the contribution that changing health may have on future rates of

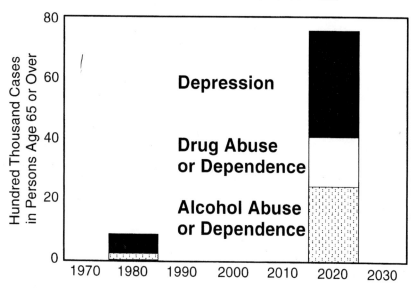

FIGURE 2.4. The Mental Health Care Crisis Ahead

Assuming increasing disability has no effect on cases of mental illness.

Source: Projected estimates compiled from data on rates of mental disorder from Reiger et al. (1988). *Archives of General Psychiatry* 45:977-986.

depression, anxiety, and substance abuse. Baby boomers have been raised during a time of unprecedented technological growth and economic prosperity, and are perhaps experiencing better health than any generation that has preceded them. As persons age, however, they often experience changes in their health with the onset and progression of chronic illness and disability. These conditions, in turn, are frequently accompanied by feelings of depression, anxiety, and helplessness (see Figure 2.5). In such circumstances, many persons turn to alcohol or drugs to numb their emotional pain (see Figure 2.6). What will happen as this segment of the population faces, for the first time, problems with physical health, economic hardships, and other losses associated

FIGURE 2.5. Relationship Between Disability and Depression

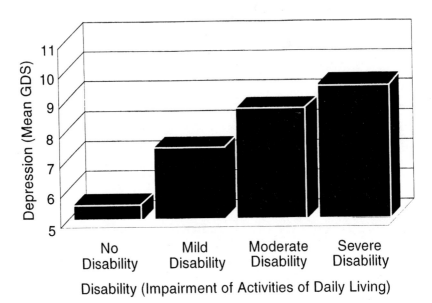

GDS = Geriatric Depression Scale; p<.001.

Source: 1987-1988 VA Mental Health Survey of 850 hospitalized patients age 65 or over, unpublished results.

FIGURE 2.6. Lifetime Alcoholism by Disability Status

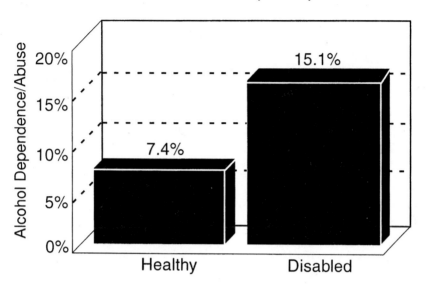

Source: Epidemiologic Catchment Area Survey (1983-1984), North Carolina site, of 2,953 adults aged 18 to 96, unpublished results.

with aging? More important, who will help them cope with these changes and provide the physical care they will need?

## *FAMILY TRENDS*

While past generations have made great efforts to care for the needs of aging parents and family members, there is concern that future generations may not be so willing or able. Three changes in the traditional American family contribute to this concern.

First, as noted before, families today are working hard to meet the economic needs required by modern lifestyles. This often requires not only that both husband and wife work outside the home, but also that they must be geographically mobile to get jobs. Consequently, adult children may find themselves living and working far away from parents and siblings. Many aging parents are now becoming geographically isolated from their adult children and losing sources of support that previous, less mobile generations had readily available. When older family members become unable to care for themselves, they often must relocate to where adult children live. Three out of ten older adults move at least once every five years.[8] With such moves, there is a loss of social support networks that may have taken nearly a half-century to develop.[9] After such a move, aging parents become increasingly dependent on adult children for both physical care and emotional sustenance. The busy lives of their adult children leave them little time for their own children, let alone their aging parents.

Second, in a society where the divorce rate nearly equals the marriage rate, single-parent homes are rapidly becoming the norm for certain segments of our population. In the year 2000, only 53 percent of families will include both a husband and a wife present.[10] Families in which the father is absent are nine times more likely than two-parent homes to have incomes of less than $10,000.[11] Consequently, many persons are moving into their later years without a spouse who can provide care for them and without the finances to pay for care themselves. Again, this puts greater pressure on children to provide for their care needs. These aging parents, however, because of work responsibilities during their own younger and middle years, may have devoted relatively little time to those adult children whom they are now expecting to care for them. Thus, a vicious cycle may develop that affects families' willingness to care for older members.

Third, members of today's society are sometimes characterized as the "me" generation, priding themselves on being independent and self-sufficient. As competition for resources increases, the focus on self and assuring that "my needs are met" becomes the modus operandi. Pop psychology often reinforces this narcissistic trend by suggesting that persons focus on meeting their own needs, as opposed to meeting the needs of others. This results in the belief that self-sacrifice and suffering are to be avoided at all cost. Persons growing up in a society with such attitudes may have little motivation to care for aging relatives, an activity which may bring little self-gratification.

These changes in the family are only trends and do not apply to all American families. Their cumulative effect, however, may be significant, and over decades and generations may have disturbing consequences, particularly in a society coming under increasing economic constraints.

## *ECONOMIC TRENDS*

Since the 1960s, government welfare programs such as Social Security, Medicare, and Medicaid have provided financial support, and physical and mental health care to the economically disadvantaged, the disabled, and the elderly. During this time, however, the government has accumulated a debt of 5.5 trillion dollars (1996), and great efforts are now being made to "balance the budget" and limit expenditures, especially expenditures for health care. This is understandable, given the astronomical increases in Medicare expenditures over the past 15 years, rocketing from 38 billion in 1980 to almost 170 billion in 1995 (see Figure 2.7). What is of particular concern is that such increases have occurred at a time *preceding* the greatest increase in the number of older persons this country has ever known (see Figure 2.1).

Reports indicate that 1995 was the first year since 1972 in which the Medicare Hospitalization Insurance Trust Fund paid out more money than it took in through payroll taxes.[12] There are predictions that the trust fund will be empty by the year 2001 or sooner.[13] At that time, our collective health bill will reach nearly 2 trillion dollars, almost one-fifth of the nation's entire economic output.[13,14] If Medicare does go broke, the Medicare trustees project that payroll taxes will increase from 2.9 percent (in 1996)

FIGURE 2.7. Federal Funding of Health Care for the Elderly

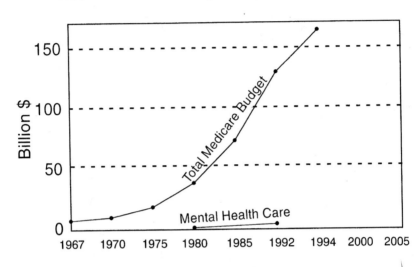

Mental health care equaled 1.5 percent of 1980 Medicare budget and 3 percent of 1992 budget.

Source: Data from Levit et al. (1996). Healthcare spending in 1994. *Health Affairs* 15(2):141.

to 6.8 percent simply to keep the Medicare hospitalization program afloat,[12] and further increases will be necessary each year as the number of older persons receiving benefits increases. This does not take into consideration the Medicare premium for physicians' services (75 percent of which comes from taxpayer dollars), which is doubling every five years.

If anything, then, in the years ahead we can expect cuts, not increases, in government programs that provide physical and mental health services to older adults. The burden of funding such care will rest squarely on the shoulders of the taxpayers of the next century, particularly the working class. Will the "baby busters"—the children of the baby boomers, sometimes called "Generation X"—be willing to tolerate such an economic drain?

## COMMUNITY RESOURCES

If funds are inadequate to support government programs that provide health care to 74 million aging baby boomers, and if family members are unavailable, unable, or unwilling to care for their aging relatives, then we are again faced with the disturbing question of who will take care of all these people. What community resources are available to prevent persons from falling through the ever-widening cracks in government-sponsored programs? Before the extensive government programs we have today, it was the church that often met the needs of the weak and vulnerable members of society.[15]

In the Middle Ages, for example, hospitals were started and staffed by clergy. At that time, *the church* was the body that issued medical licenses to physicians, many of whom were priests. Until after the French Revolution, as late as the eighteenth century, the church largely controlled medicine and the delivery of health care. After a series of corrupt Popes and church-sponsored atrocities (burning of mentally-ill elderly women as witches, to name one), the health care system finally broke free from the church's control. Even today, however, many nursing homes and hospitals in the United States and around the world are sponsored by religious bodies that have made care of the sick a primary part of their mission. In the years ahead, we may see the church taking a larger and larger role in meeting the mental and even physical health needs of aging persons.

## SUMMARY

Changes are occurring in our society. Aging baby boomers and improvements in health care are causing a rapid increase in the number of older persons in the United States. People are not necessarily surviving longer as healthy and independent individuals, however. Many aging persons experience increased disability and chronic illness. These conditions are often associated with depression, anxiety, and substance abuse. Even now, baby boomers have high rates of these disorders at a time when they are generally healthy and economically well off. There is reason to worry about the future mental health of this generation as they face the physical, social, and economic losses of aging. In particular, there is concern about who will provide the physical and mental health care that this 74-million-member cohort will require, given changes in family structure and values, as well as increasing financial limitations to government programs that provide health care services. Should we look toward religion or religious bodies as potential sources of help for the troubling times ahead? Let us examine the arguments of health professionals who believe that we should stay clear of religion, if not discourage it.

## REFERENCE NOTES

1. National Center for Health Statistics. (1990). *Health, United States, 1989 and Prevention Profile.* DHHS Pub. No. (PHS) 90-1232. Hyattsville, MD: U.S. Department of Health and Human Services.

2. *Healthy People 2000.* (1991). National Health Promotion and Disease Prevention: U.S. Department of Health and Human Services, Public Health Service, DHHS Publication No. (PHS) 91-50212.

3. Spencer, G. (1989). Projections of the population of the United States, by age, sex, and race: 1988 to 2080. *Current Population Reports, Population Estimates and Projections.* Series P-25, No. 1018. Washington, DC: U.S. Department of Commerce, Bureau of the Census.

4. Schick and Schick. (1994). *Statistical Handbook on Aging Americans* (Series #5). New York: Oryx Press.

5. Kunkel, S.R., and R.A. Applebaum. (1992). Estimating the prevalence of long-term disability for an aging society. *Journal of Gerontology* (Social Sciences) 47:S253-S260.

6. Evans, D.A., H.H. Funkenstein, M.S. Albert, P.A. Scherr, N.R. Cook, M.J. Chown, L.E. Hebert, C.H. Hennekens, and J.O. Taylor. (1989). Prevalence of Alzheimer's disease in a community population of older persons. Higher than previously reported. *Journal of the American Medical Association* 262:2551-2556.

7. Regier, D.A., J.H. Boyd, J.D. Burke, D.S. Rae, J.K. Myers, M. Kramer, L.N. Robins, L.K. George, M. Karno, and B.Z. Locke. (1988). One-month preva-

lence of mental disorders in the United States. *Archives of General Psychiatry* 45:977-986.

8. Flynn, C.B., C.F. Longino, R.F. Wiseman, and J.C. Biggar. (1985). The redistribution of America's older population: Major national migration patterns for three census decades, 1960-1980. *The Gerontologist* 25:292-296.

9. Coffman, T.L. (1987). Relocation and relocation stress. In G.L. Maddox (Ed.), *The Encyclopedia of Aging.* NY: Springer Publishing Co.

10. Bureau of the Census. *Projections of the Numbers of Households and Families: 1986 to 2000.* Washington, DC: U.S. Department of Commerce.

11. U.S. Congress, House Select Committee on Children, Youth, and Families. *U.S. Children and their Families: Current Conditions and Recent Trends.* Washington, DC: The Congress.

12. Moffit, R.E. (1996). Generation X and the Medicare bills. Editorial (Scripps Howard), *The Durham Herald-Sun* (March 11, 1996), p. A9.

13. Associated Press. (1993). Medicare trust fund going broke. Fund could be drained by 1998. *The Durham Herald-Sun* (April 7, 1993), p. 3.

14. Associated Press. (1994). Report moves up depletion of Social Security by 8 years. *The Durham Herald-Sun* (April 12, 1994), p. A7.

15. Kuhn, C.C. (1988). A spiritual inventory of the medically ill patient. *Psychiatric Medicine* 6:87-100.

# Chapter 3

# Negative Effects of Religion on Health

Might religion *not* be good for health? According to a substantial number of mental health professionals, this is precisely the case. It has been argued that religion has a neurotic influence that breeds mental inflexibility, emotional instability, and unhealthy repression of natural instincts. At best, most medical doctors see religion as harmless but largely irrelevant to health or health care, and religious issues are usually not addressed during a medical visit unless they interfere with medical treatment (for example, a Jehovah's Witness refusing blood transfusions). There is a range of opinions that leading health professionals have expressed about religion over the years. Let's examine them now.

## *SIGMUND FREUD*

Almost 60 years ago, Freud–considered the father of modern psychiatry–argued convincingly that religion was linked with neurosis. So concerned about the subject, he spent most of the last ten years of his life writing about religion's neurotic influences on mental health.[1-4] In *Future of an Illusion*,[5] Freud rationalized that religion was a neurotic vestige of the Oedipal complex, and that therapy would reduce the need for religion and replace it with more conscious and emotionally healthy processes:

> Religion would thus be the universal obsessional neurosis of humanity; like the obsessional neurosis of children, it

arose out of the Oedipus complex, out of the relation to the father. . . . Historical residues have helped us to view religious teachings, as it were, as neurotic relics, and we may now argue that the time has probably come, as it does in analytic treatment, for replacing the effects of repression by the results of the rational operation of the intellect. (pp. 43-44)

and

Our God, Logos [human reason], will fulfill whichever of these wishes nature outside us allows, but will do it very gradually, only in the unforeseeable future, and for a new generation of man. He promises noncompensation for us, who suffer grievously from life. On the way to this distant goal your religious doctrines will have to be discarded, no matter whether the first attempts fail or whether the first substitutes prove untenable. And you know why: in the long run nothing can withstand reason and experience, and the contradiction which religion offers to both is all too palpable. (p. 54)

While Freud rejected traditional religious beliefs of his day, he was in private a superstitious man. Freud was obsessed with death and preoccupied with certain numbers (especially the number 17) as a way of predicting good luck and foretelling the date of his own death. After declining an invitation to speak at the American Psychical Institute in 1921, Freud wrote, "If I were at the beginning of a scientific career, instead of, as now, at its end, I would perhaps choose no other field of work [than parapsychology] in spite of all the difficulties."[6]

Freud's negative attitudes toward traditional religious beliefs and practices have had widespread effects on the mental health field. The message to his colleagues and students was that belief in God served no healthy purpose and could be dispensed with.

While Freud sometimes claimed there was no conflict between religion and his technique of psychoanalysis, in practice this was often not the case. Writing in a major psychiatric journal of the day, O. Fenichel[7]–a leading psychoanalyst in the generation following Freud–stated

> It has been said that religious people in analysis remain uninfluenced in their religious philosophies since analysis itself is supposed to be philosophically neutral. I consider this not to be correct. Repeatedly I have seen that with the analysis of the sexual anxieties and with maturing of the personality, the attachment to religion has ended. (p. 89)

## *ALBERT ELLIS*

Dr. Ellis, founder and president of the Rational Emotive Therapy Institute in New York, is best known for his contributions to the development of cognitive-behavioral therapy–perhaps the most widely used psychotherapeutic technique for treating depression, anxiety, and other emotional disorders. Ellis wrote the following comment in a 1980 issue of the *Journal of Consulting and Clinical Psychology*, the flagship journal for the American Psychological Association:[8]

> Devout, orthodox, or dogmatic religion (or what might be called religiosity) is significantly correlated with emotional disturbance. People largely disturb themselves by believing strongly in absolutistic shoulds, oughts, and musts, and most people who dogmatically believe in some religion believe in these health-sabotaging absolutes. The emotionally healthy individual is flexible, open, tolerant, and changing, and the devoutly religious person tends to be inflexible, closed, intolerant, and unchanging. Religiosity, therefore, is in many respects equivalent to irrational thinking and emotional disturbance. (p. 637)

Ellis reiterated and expanded these views more recently in the journal *Free Inquiry* asking the question, "Is religiosity pathological?"[9] He identified 11 characteristics of religiosity that run counter to sound mental health. These characteristics included the following:

- Discouragement of self-acceptance, self-interest, and self-directedness;
- Promotion of intolerance of others, inflexibility, and the inability to deal with ambiguity and uncertainty–all of which impact negatively on human-to-human relationships;
- Encouragement of a reliance on God, the ignoring of reality, and the discouragement of individual actions necessary for problem resolution;
- Promotion of fanatical commitments; and
- Discouragement of appropriate risk-taking in pursuit of personal goals.

Ellis concludes that an irrefutable causal relationship exists between religion and emotional and mental illness. When asked recently about his opinion concerning recent research demonstrating a positive influence of religion on health, he responded, "This whole field is off its rocker . . . These studies should not be taken too seriously."[10] The discussion in Chapters 5 and 6 explores just how seriously this research should be taken.

## WENDELL WATTERS

Dr. Watters is a respected physician and professor of psychiatry at McMaster University in Ontario, Canada, and a psychoanalyst who has treated individuals, couples, and families for over a quarter of a century. In 1992, he published a book titled *Deadly Doctrine* (Prometheus Books). In the introduction, he writes the following:[11]

The thesis of this book, based on many years of clinical experience, is that despite the so-called comfort of the Christian message, Christian doctrine and teachings, deeply ingrained as they are in Western society, are incompatible with the development and maintenance of sound health, and not only 'mental' health, in human beings . . . Simply put, Christian indoctrination is a form of mental and emotional abuse that can adversely affect bodily health in the same way a drug can. . . . However, evidence that religion is not only irrelevant but actually harmful to human beings should be of interest, not only to other behavioral scientists, but to anyone who finds it difficult to live an unexamined life. Finally, the argument advanced in this volume should stir the political decision makers who complain about the high costs of health care even while continuing to subsidize that very institution that may be actually making the public 'sick.' (pp. 10,12)

Dr. Watters moves on to explain how religious teachings might play an important role in the genesis of specific mental illnesses such as schizophrenia, depression, and other major psychiatric disorders, emphasizing that Christian doctrine and teachings are incompatible with the primary components of sound mental health, particularly self-esteem, self-actualization and mastery; good communication skills, "related individuation," and establishment of supportive social networks; and the development of healthy sexuality (p. 140).

## OTHER MENTAL HEALTH PROFESSIONALS

In the third edition of the American Psychiatric Association's *Diagnostic and Statistical Manual of Mental Disorders* (*DSM-III-R*), religion is consistently portrayed in a negative light. In fact, 12 references to religion in the Glossary of Technical Terms are used to illustrate psychopathology.[12] (This is now changed in the new *DSM-IV*, which uses terminology that is more sensitive to the religious or cultural backgrounds and experiences of patients.) Remarking on the current state of affairs in psychology, noted Yale psychologist Seymour B. Sarason[13] stated the following in his 1992 centennial address before the American Psychological Association:

> I think I am safe in assuming that the bulk of the membership of the American Psychological Association would, if asked, describe themselves as agnostic or atheistic. I am also safe in assuming that any one or all of the ingredients of the religious world view are of neither personal nor professional interest to most psychologists. . . . Indeed, if we learn that someone is devoutly religious, or even tends in that direction, we look upon that person with puzzlement, often concluding that psychologist obviously had or has personal problems.

Thus, it appears that many prominent mental health professionals of the twentieth century believe that religion has either no influence on mental health or a negative one.

## PRIMARY CARE PHYSICIANS

The views of family physicians and internists toward religion have been less hostile than those of mental health professionals. They have not, however, been particularly warm to the topic, nor has there been any substantive attempt to include religion as a component of clinical care. Several years ago, geriatric medicine specialist Nina Covalt addressed the topic of religion and health care in the widely circulated medical journal, *Geriatrics*. Dr. Covalt wrote that she had not observed elderly people asking for more spiritual help when they were ill, and that during her 25 years of medical practice, no patients ever approached her to discuss religious beliefs or problems or even to ask for a minister.[14] In fact, she reported, it was a sign of trouble for the physician if a sick patient brought a Bible along with them to the hospital and kept it displayed at the bedside.

There is even more resistance from the medical community when it comes to "faith healing," though this resistance may be applied more generally to various traditional religious beliefs and practices as well. For example, response from the medical community was largely negative to an editorial that appeared in the prominent British medical journal *Lancet* which reviewed past research on faith healing.[15] The article also discussed the work and future research of Great Britain's Confederation of Healing Organizations, which represents over 7,000 healers from a wide variety of persuasions. Many in the medical community expressed concern about the dangers that could result from faith healing, particularly the stopping of medications.[16]

Faith healing (as seen in tent revivals), however, is advocated by only a small proportion of the Judeo-Christian faith community in the United States. More common is the belief that a person's faith and prayer can contribute to their healing on many levels, even if not by a dramatic outward manifestation of sudden, complete cure (as typically sought by faith healers). One study of 586 adults randomly sampled by telephone discovered that 14 percent had experienced divine healing of a serious disease or physical condition.[17]. Despite patients' beliefs about their religion's potential impact on health, a significant number of physicians continue to believe that religious issues of this or any kind should not be discussed during a medical visit, and some do not even refer patients who raise religious issues to clergy for help.[18] When patients themselves are asked, between two-thirds and three-quarters indicate that their physicians never address religious issues with them.[19]

## *SUMMARY*

A significant number of mental health experts have argued that religious beliefs and practices are neurotic, maladaptive, and foster the development of guilt, depression, and other mental disorders. These individuals have strongly influenced the mental health field in its attitude toward religion. Primary care physicians and other medical professionals, while less forceful in their negative opinions of religion's influences than their psychiatric colleagues, nevertheless largely see religion as irrelevant to health and the delivery of good health care. Let us now examine how common and influential religious beliefs and practices are in the United States today, as we further seek to determine whether traditional religious beliefs and practices have positive, negative, or neutral effects on health.

## REFERENCE NOTES

1. Freud, S. (1930). *Civilization and Its Discontents.* Standard Edition, London: Hogarth Press, 1962.

2. Freud, S. (1933). *Why War?* Standard Edition, London: Hogarth Press, 1962.

3. Freud, S. (1933). *New Introductory Lectures.* Standard Edition, London: Hogarth Press, 1962.

4. Freud, S. (1939). *Moses and Monotheism.* Standard Edition, London: Hogarth Press, 1962.

5. Freud, S. (1927). *Future of an Illusion.* Standard Edition, London: Hogarth Press, 1962.

6. Wallace, E.R. (1978). Freud's mysticism and its psychodynamic determinants. *Bulletin of the Menninger Clinic* 42:210-222.

7. Fenichel, O. (1941). *Problems of Psychoanalytic Technique.* NY: Psychoanalytic Quarterly.

8. Ellis, A. (1980). Psychotherapy and atheistic values: A response to A.E. Bergin's "Psychotherapy and religious values." *Journal of Consulting and Clinical Psychology* 48:642-645.

9. Ellis, A. (1988). Is religiosity pathological? *Free Inquiry* 18:27-32.

10. Ellis, A. (1996). *USA Weekend* (April 5-7, 1996), p. 4.

11. Watters, Wendell, W., MD (1992). *Deadly Doctrine: Health, Illness, and Christian God-Talk.* Amherst, NY: Prometheus Books. Reprinted by permission of the publisher.

12. Larson, D.B., S.B. Thielman, M.A. Greenwold, J.S. Lyons, S.G. Post, K.A. Sherrill, G.G. Wood, and S.S. Larson. (1993). Religious content in the DSM-III-R glossary of technical terms. *American Journal of Psychiatry* 150:1884-1885.

13. Sarason, S.B. (1992). Centennial Address. 1992 Annual Meeting of the American Psychological Association.

14. Covalt, N. (1960). The meaning of religion to older people. *Geriatrics* 15:658-664.

15. *Lancet*. (1985). Exploring the effectiveness of healing (editorial). (November 23, 1985), pp. 1177-1178.

16. Coakley, D.V., and G.W. McKenna. (1986). Safety of faith healing. *Lancet* (February 22, 1986), p. 444; See also Smith, D.M. (1986). Safety of faith healing. *Lancet* (March 15, 1986), p. 621.

17. Johnson, D.M., J.S. Williams, and D.G. Bromley. (1986). Religion, health, and healing: findings from a southern city. *Sociological Analysis* 47:66-73.

18. Koenig, H.G., L.B. Bearon, and R. Dayringer. (1989). Physician perspectives on the role of religion in the physician/older patient relationship. *Journal of Family Practice* 28:441-448.

19. King, D.E., and B. Bushwick. (1994). Beliefs and attitudes of hospital inpatients about faith healing and prayer. *Journal of Family Practice* 39:349-352.

Chapter 4

# Are Americans Becoming Less Religious?

There has been much discussion over the past 30 years about the secularization of society and the decline of religious influence, belief, and participation in America. Recall that Freud predicted such a decline almost three-quarters of a century ago. As scientific progress has occurred, have we become more rational and emotionally stable, and have we achieved greater control over our destiny? Are persons today more able to cope with their problems through rational means, without the aid of religious beliefs and practices, which, as Freud, Ellis, and Watters have suggested, breed emotional instability and neurosis?

## *RELIGIOUS BELIEFS*

Despite opinions to the contrary, the vast majority of Americans still believe in God or some higher power. A December 1994 Gallup Poll[1] found that 94 percent of younger Americans (ages 18 to 29) believe in God and 97 percent of older adults (ages 50 or over) do so (see Figure 4.1). The figure for all ages in both 1944 and 1996 was 96 percent.[1,2] Thus, it appears that belief in God in the United States has remained relatively stable over the past 50 years, and is among the highest of any country in the world[3] (see Figure 4.2). Compared to the general public, however, belief in God by psychologists and psychiatrists is low (43 percent and 40 to 70 percent, respectively).[4,5]

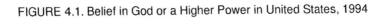

FIGURE 4.1. Belief in God or a Higher Power in United States, 1994

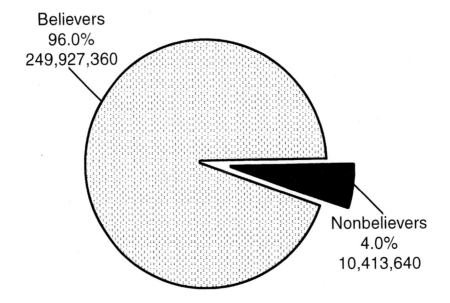

**Believers**
**96.0%**
**249,927,360**

Nonbelievers
4.0%
10,413,640

Source: Princeton Religion Research Center (December 1994). Gallup Poll.

Besides belief in God, other traditional Christian beliefs remain prevalent in this country. For many health professionals, the belief in Satan or hell seems preposterous, something that should be relegated to fairy tales, and certainly not appropriate for mature adults. Nevertheless, almost two-thirds of the American public (65 percent) continue to believe in the devil, and almost three-quarters (73 percent) believe in hell[1]; in fact, almost one-quarter (23 percent) of Americans say their chances of going to hell are good or fair. On the other hand, a much greater proportion (90 percent) believe in the existence of heaven and claim that their chances of getting there are pretty good (77 percent). Interestingly, belief in the devil and hell was *less common* among older adults. Only 57 percent of persons age 65 or over believe in the devil, compared with 69 percent under age 50. Likewise,

FIGURE 4.2. Belief in God or a Universal Spirit Worldwide

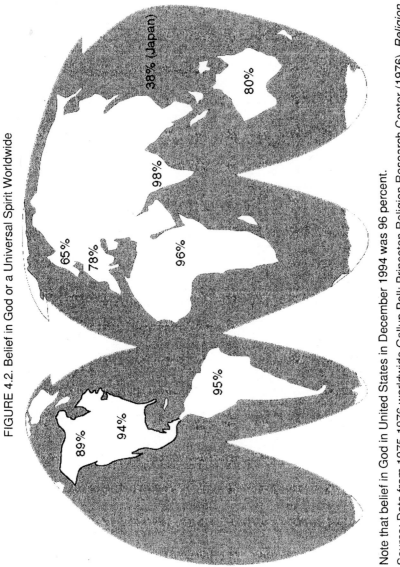

65%
78%
98%
38% (Japan)
96%
80%
89%
94%
95%

Note that belief in God in United States in December 1994 was 96 percent.

Source: Data from 1975-1976 worldwide Gallup Poll: Princeton Religion Research Center (1976). *Religion in America.* Princeton, NJ.

64 percent of those over age 65 believe in hell, compared with 75 percent of those under age 50.

In addition, many Americans believe in miracles (79 percent) and angels (72 percent), and a much smaller proportion believe in reincarnation (27 percent) or astrology (23 percent). Finally, 84 percent of Americans believe that Jesus is God or the son of God.[1] In a country known for its education, communication of knowledge, and progress in science and rational thought, religious beliefs remain widely prevalent.

## *IMPORTANCE OF RELIGION*

While religious beliefs may be common, how important are these beliefs? A 1995 Gallup Poll[1] found that 58 percent of Americans indicated that religion was very important in their lives (45 percent of persons under age 30 and 73 percent of those over age 65). Only 9 percent indicated that it was not important. Note that since 1978 (when 52 percent said religion was very important) there has been relatively little change, although it is less than in 1952 when 75 percent said it was very important.[6] How important is religion to Americans, compared to persons in other countries around the world? An international study found that only South Africans exceed Americans in ratings of "importance of God in life."[2] This particular survey, however, did not include India or the Muslim countries.

## *INFLUENCE OF RELIGION ON LIFE*

In 1982, Gallup Polls[7] asked Americans to respond to the statement "My religious faith is the most important influence in my life." Sixty-nine percent of respondents (84 percent of older adults) indicated that this was "completely true" or "mostly true," whereas only 10 percent said that it was "completely untrue."

There has been a widespread perception over the past decade, however, that religion is losing its influence in this country. In 1985, Gallup Polls found that 49 percent of surveyed respondents thought that religion was increasing influence and 39 percent thought that it was losing influence in American life.[8] If one looks at Gallup Poll results from over 50 years ago (1939), the figures were 30 percent for gaining influence and 34 percent for losing influence.[9] Thus, people's perceptions had changed relatively little during the nearly 50 years between these polls. While no national surveys since 1982 have asked Americans to respond to the statement "My religious faith is the most important influence in my life," Gallup Polls have asked on a yearly basis whether religion is gaining or losing influence in American life. The latter question is a different one from the former question, however, because it does not assess the personal influence that religion has on people's lives, rather only their perceptions about religion's influence in the world around them. Over the past ten years the percentage of Americans saying that religion's influence on American life is decreasing has increased from 39 percent in 1985 to 57 percent in 1995.[1]

## *RELIGIOUS AFFILIATION*

When we talk about "religion" in this country, what do we mean? Most Americans are affiliated with Christian denominations. In June 1994,[10] 85 percent of Americans were affiliated with Protestant (61 percent) or Catholic (24 percent) denominations, whereas 2 percent were Mormon, 2 percent Jewish, 5 percent other (including 1 percent Greek or Russian Orthodox and less than 1 percent affiliated with Hindu or Muslim faith traditions). Among Protestants, the largest groups were Baptist (22 percent), Methodist (9 percent), Lutheran (7 percent), Presbyterian (4 percent), Episcopal (2 percent), Pentecostal/Assembly of God (2 percent), nondenominational (6 percent), and other (7 percent) (see Figure 4.3). The percentage of Americans with no religious affiliation, however, has increased from a low of 2 percent in 1967 to a high of 11 percent in 1990.[11] Age differences are particularly notable in this regard. In 1992 and 1993, only 5 percent of persons age 50 or over had no religious preference, compared with 10 percent of those ages 30 to 49 and 13 percent of those under age 30.[6] Many congregations, indeed, are aging. By the year 2000, over 50 percent of the members of mainline Protestant denominations will be over the age of 60[6] (see Figure 4.4). This epidemiologic fact underscores how important it is that mainline Protestant traditions pay increasing attention to the particular emotional and spiritual needs of persons in this age group.

## *CHURCH MEMBERSHIP*

In 1937, 73 percent of Americans said they were members of churches or synagogues.[2] In 1994, the figure was 70 percent.[10] While only 61 percent of persons under age 30 were members in a church or synagogue in 1994, 80 percent of those over age 65 were.[1] As with other indicators of religiousness, the proportion of the population claiming church membership has not changed much over the years. One of the reasons why older adults are more likely to be church members is that this generation is known for its pro-institutional stance, whereas more recent generations born since World War II have tended to be anti-institutional. Nevertheless, as these persons age, they are establishing their own institutions (which their children are likely to rebel against, just as they did).

## *CHURCH ATTENDANCE*

In 1995, 43 percent of Americans attended church or synagogue at least once within the past seven days; the figure increased

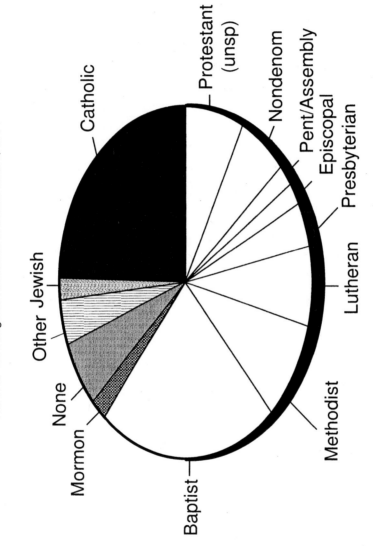

FIGURE 4.3. Religious Affiliations in United States, 1994

FIGURE 4.4. Projected Percent of Members Age 60 or Over, of Selected Religions, in the Year 2000

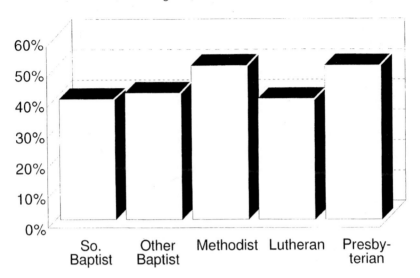

Source: Projected from Princeton Religion Research Center (1994 Supplement). Gallup Poll, 1992-1993.

to 53 percent for persons age 65 or over.[1] This makes religious participation the most common form of voluntary group social activity in the United States. In fact, if one combines all other forms of voluntary group activity, it still does not exceed involvement in church. To what extent has religious participation declined over the past 50 years? In 1939, 41 percent of Americans attended church at least weekly; in 1950, 39 percent did so; in 1967, 43 percent did so; and in 1980, the figure was 40 percent[2,6] (see Figure 4.5). Thus, there has been almost no change in the proportion of Americans attending church since the death of Freud in 1939.

This is true in general for involvement in organized religion. Based on a Princeton Religion Research Center Index (composed of factors such as belief in God; confidence in religion, church

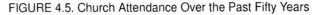

FIGURE 4.5. Church Attendance Over the Past Fifty Years

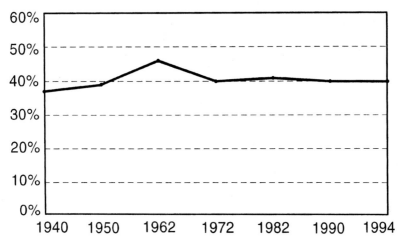

Percent of respondents who attended church/synagogue in last seven days.

Source: Princeton Religion Research Center (1940-1994). Gallup Polls.

and clergy; and church membership and preference levels), the importance of organized religion in the United States today is only slightly lower than it was in the 1940s. On this index, Americans achieved a point score of 733 in the 1940s compared with 665 in 1996. Interestingly, the 1996 score is the highest it has been in 10 years.[1]

The following comparison gives us a good sense of America's religious involvement. Given the avid attention paid by Americans to sporting events, one might surely think that attendance at sporting events would exceed that of church. According to research done by the late George Cornell, well-known Associated Press writer, and the Gallup organization, this is simply not true. Americans spent four billion dollars on sporting events in 1992, compared with *57 billion dollars* donated to religious causes. In 1993, attendance at all professional baseball, football, and basketball games numbered 103 million; yearly attendance at both professional and college football, baseball, hockey, basketball, boxing, tennis, soccer, wrestling; and harness, auto, and dog racing, increases the figure to 388 million (1990 estimate). Compare this with *over 5 billion visits* per year to local churches and synagogues in 1990 (see Figure 4.6).

Recent information from a survey by George Barna suggests that church attendance in this country may have declined some since 1991, particularly among baby boomers. The Barna survey[12] examined beliefs and attitudes of 1,004 adults in the United States in 1995. While 82 percent of Americans in the sample called themselves religious, only 37 percent reported attending worship services in the past week (compared to 40 percent in 1991); persons born between 1946 and 1964 had the lowest rates of weekly church attendance (31 percent), even lower than the 34 percent of baby busters (ages 18 to 30) who worshipped in the past week.

FIGURE 4.6. Which Is More Important to Americans: Sports or Religion?

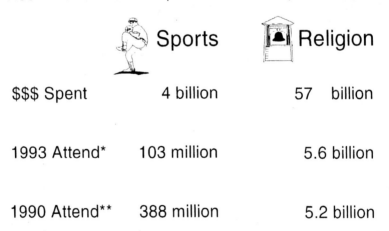

| | Sports | Religion |
| --- | --- | --- |
| $$$ Spent | 4 billion | 57   billion |
| 1993 Attend* | 103 million | 5.6 billion |
| 1990 Attend** | 388 million | 5.2 billion |

*Professional baseball, football, and basketball.
**Both professional and college football, baseball, hockey, basketball, boxing, tennis, soccer, wrestling; and harness, auto, and dog racing.

Source: Cornell, George (1992), Associated Press Writer, and Gallup Poll (1994).

As usual, persons age 50 or older attended church most often (50 percent).

## *RELIGIOUS TELEVISION*

One would expect that after all the scandals concerning tele-vangelists over the past decade, Americans would have been turned off to religious TV programs. Not so. According to a 1987 Gallup Poll[8] taken after the fall of Jim Baker, Americans actually increased their watching of religious TV from 42 percent in 1983 to 49 percent in 1987. In fact, 25 percent had watched religious TV within the past seven days (compared with 18 percent in 1983) and an additional 24 percent within the past month (same in 1983). Almost two-thirds of older adults (64 percent) watch religious TV. Much fewer Americans actually contribute money to TV evangelists, although there is a relationship with age. Less than 1 percent of persons under age 30 contribute, whereas 7 per-cent of those over age 50 do so. Many older adults with health problems that limit their mobility watch religious TV or listen to religious radio to compensate for not being able to attend church.

## *PRAYER*

Ninety percent of Americans say they pray. When asked how they pray, 87 percent indicate they pray silently or alone, whereas 11 percent pray aloud or with others.[6] Over 95 percent of persons age 50 or older pray. Of those who pray, 97 percent believe their prayers are heard and 95 percent believe their prayers have been answered. What do they pray about? Ninety-eight percent pray for their family's well-being, 94 percent offer prayers of thanks, and 92 percent pray for strength or guidance to meet a challenge. Only a few (5 percent) pray for something bad to happen to someone else.[1] What types of prayers are Americans saying? Fifty-six percent pray in a personal or conversational manner, 15 percent pray in a meditative or reflective manner, 13 percent pray formally (such as the Lord's Prayer), and 14 percent do a combination of all three. Of those who pray, only 1 percent say that prayer is less important to them now than it was five years ago.[1]

## BIBLE READING

According to a November 1990 Gallup Poll, 80 percent of Americans read the Bible.[13] Forty percent read the Bible at least weekly (52 percent of those are over age 50). What do Americans believe about the Bible? Almost one-third (31 percent) believe the Bible is the *actual word* of God and is to be taken literally. Another quarter (24 percent) believe the Bible is the *inspired word* of God, that it contains no errors, but that some verses are to be taken symbolically rather than literally. Thus, over one-half of persons in this country believe that the Bible is either the literal or inspired word of God and contains no errors. Fifty-five percent of Americans indicate they have read most or all of the New Testament, whereas 44 percent say they have read most or all of the Old Testament. What proportion of Americans belong to a Bible study group? In 1978, 19 percent belonged to Bible study groups, compared to 26 percent in 1985 and 21 percent in 1990.

## RELIGION AND AGING

We have seen that for virtually every category of religious belief and activity, older persons are more involved than younger persons. There has been debate about why this is so. Has today's generation of older adults always been more religious (even when younger), or did they become that way as they grew older?

In other words, does interest in religion remain constant with age or does it increase in importance as people age? While it is likely that today's generation of older Americans grew up during a period when religion had greater influence on society and the family (called a "cohort effect"), this is probably not the entire explanation. There is mounting evidence that aging itself may affect a person's interest in religion. Existential concerns at this time in life might prompt aging persons to reexamine their views about God or perhaps adopt a religious worldview to help cope with stress and life change.

Our research group at Duke recently asked several hundred younger and older hospitalized patients if religion had become more important to them, less important, or had stayed about the same as they had grown older.[14] The majority said that it had increased in importance with age. They related this increase to a wide variety of causes including health changes, recovery from an addiction or alcoholism, or the influence of family members or friends. Only about 5 percent indicated that religion's importance had decreased with age.

Furthermore, surveys of the American public during the 1940s by the Gallup organization found the same age pattern of interest in religion that we see today. Over 50 years ago, younger persons were less religious than older persons. A 1944 poll conducted by the American Institute of Public Opinion[15] reported that 93 percent of persons aged 20 to 29 believed in God, compared with 97 percent of those over age 50. Similarly, 70 percent of persons aged 20 to 29 reported that they believed in an afterlife, compared with 79 percent of those over age 50. In 1949, persons were asked whether people in this country would go to church more or less often in the next 50 years than they did then. Forty percent of persons age 20 to 29 said less often compared with 28 percent of those over age 50 who said less often.[16] In 1942, 48 percent of persons aged 20 to 29 read the Bible in the past year, compared with 58 percent of those aged 30 to 49 and 71 percent of those aged 50 or over.[9] Thus, while a "cohort effect" may be operative to some extent, it cannot by itself explain the greater religiousness of older Americans today.

## SUMMARY

Religion continues to play an important role in the lives of Americans of every age. Religious belief and activity are lowest among baby boomers and young adults, and highest among those who are older. There is some evidence that as persons grow older and more experienced–particularly after facing traumatic, uncontrollable life stresses–they may become more religious. In general, there is little indication that religious belief or activity has become unimportant to the vast majority of citizens of the most educated, scientifically sophisticated, technologically advanced nation in the world–quite contrary to Freud's predictions. Why would religion persist in such a widespread and extensive manner in this country if its effects on mental and physical health were as damaging and destructive as argued in Chapter 3? In the next chapter, we will take an objective look at the relationship between religion and mental health.

## REFERENCE NOTES

1. Princeton Religion Research Center. (1996). *Religion in America: Will the vitality of the church be the surprise of the 21st century?* Princeton, NJ: Gallup Poll.

2. Princeton Religion Research Center. (1985). *Religion in America: 50 years: 1935-1985*. Princeton, NJ: Gallup Poll (report #236).

3. Princeton Religion Research Center. (1976). *Religion in America.* Princeton, NJ: Gallup Poll.

4. Ragan, C., H.N. Malony, and B. Beit-Hallahmi. (1980). Psychologists and religion: Professional factors and personal belief. *Review of Religious Research* 21:208-217.

5. American Psychiatric Association. (1975). *Task Force Report 10: Psychiatrists' Viewpoints on Religion and Their Services to Religious Institutions and the Ministry.* Washington, DC: APA.

6. Princeton Religion Research Center. (1994). *Emerging Trends* 16 (1):1. Princeton, NJ: Gallup Poll.

7. Princeton Religion Research Center. (1982). *Religion in America.* Princeton, NJ: Gallup Poll.

8. Princeton Religion Research Center. (1987). *Religion in America.* Princeton, NJ: Gallup Poll.

9. American Institute of Public Opinion. (1939 and 1942). Princeton, NJ: The Gallup Poll.

10. Gallup Poll News Service. (1995). *Religious Trends.* Princeton Religious Research Center, Princeton, NJ.

11. Princeton Religion Research Center. (1990). *Emerging Trends.* Princeton, NJ: Gallup Poll.

12. Religion News Service. Boomers drop churchgoing to a new low. *The Durham Herald-Sun,* pp. B1-B2, March 9, 1996.

13. Princeton Religion Research Center. (1990). *The Role of the Bible in American Society.* Princeton, NJ: Gallup Poll.

14. Koenig, H.G. (1994). *Aging and God.* Binghamton, NY: The Haworth Press.

15. American Institute of Public Opinion. (1944). Princeton, NJ: The Gallup Poll.

16. American Institute of Public Opinion. (1949). Princeton, NJ: The Gallup Poll.

# Chapter 5

# Religion and Mental Health

Do traditional religious beliefs and practices foster mental illness, neurosis, depression, and perhaps schizophrenia? The arguments made by Freud, Ellis, and Watters are largely based on anecdotal case reports, "clinical experience," and most often, personal opinion. Of course, the same holds true for claims to the contrary by clergy and religious professionals. Today, however, we have another method to help settle this dispute–the scientific method. While this is certainly a less-than-perfect method for determining the truth, particularly when studying vague and difficult-to-measure concepts like mental health and religiousness, still this method represents an advance over personal experience or a heavily biased selection of cases that support one's worldview. Thus, systematic scientific research allows us to move beyond the personal debate between religious and health professionals to a more objective realm–not completely devoid of bias or error, but at least less subjective than previous strategies. With systematic research, the findings speak for themselves.

During the past half-century, especially the last ten years, a number of well-designed studies have examined the relationship between mental health and religious belief, commitment, or practice. We will review some of this research.

I have chosen to focus primarily on the work done at Duke University Medical Center over the past ten to 15 years, and to discuss the studies by other investigators as they relate to the disorders we have been studying here. Readers wishing a more comprehensive review of the literature on mental health and religion are referred to the General Reviews of the Research Literature section at the back of this book.

## *RELIGIOUS COPING*

The first step in assessing religion's impact on mental health is to simply ask people, as I did during my early clinical practice, whether religion helps them to cope with stress. When such studies are done, between 85 percent and 90 percent of persons respond that religion is a source of comfort.[1,2] This high percentage of affirmative responses, however, may partly result from the fact that saying "yes" to a question about religion providing comfort is a *socially desirable response*. In other words, regardless of their experience with religion, some persons may say that it comforts them because this is the "right" response, the one they think the interviewer is expecting.

A more valid way of assessing whether religion is truly a coping resource is to ask an open-ended question without mentioning religion. Instead of "Does religion help you to cope?" the interviewer might ask "What enables you to cope with the difficult or stressful events in your life?" Here, respondents must think carefully and come up with whatever activity they believe helps them. In studies that have used this technique, between 20 percent and 45 percent of persons bring up the subject of religion (prayer, God, church, etc.).[3-5] This is especially true for persons facing serious health problems or those in the midst of severe life stress.

Our research group recently surveyed 298 consecutively admitted patients to the general medical services at Duke University Medical Center, asking them questions about how they coped with life-threatening physical illness. Even before the interviewer began asking specific questions about the role of religion, over 40 percent of the patients brought up the subject;

"the Lord," "prayer," "faith in God," and so forth, were spontaneous responses to the open-ended question "What enables you to cope?" The interviewer then asked the specific question of whether religion was used to cope with the stress of their illnesses, and asked patients to rate on a scale from 0 to 10 the extent to which they used religious belief or activity to cope. Figure 5.1 shows patients' responses to that question.[5] Almost 90 percent indicated that they used religion at least to a "moderate" extent (5 or higher); 60 percent indicated at least to a large extent (7.5 or higher); and 40 percent ranked religion at 10 (the most important factor that enabled them to cope).

Thus, four out of ten randomly selected patients admitted to the medical services of a tertiary-care teaching hospital indicated that religion is *the most important factor* (more so than even family or friends) that enabled them to cope. It is hard to imagine that these religious beliefs (over 95 percent Christian) were as Wendell Watters writes, "incompatible with many of the components of sound mental health" (p. 140, *Deadly Doctrine*). Indeed, most of these patients had no mental illness whatsoever and, if anything, were coping remarkably well with some very difficult health problems. (In general, the more severe the stressor and less controllable it was, the more likely it was that people would turn to religion for comfort.) For example, in studies of hospitalized patients, we found that as the severity of the medical illness increased, religion was increasingly used as a coping behavior[6] (see Figure 5.2).

Just because people claim that religion helps them cope does not necessarily mean that it actually does so. Alcoholics often maintain that smoking cigarettes and drinking help them cope better with their nerves; clearly, however, these coping behaviors in the long run do not enhance health, increase well-being, or reduce depression. Thus, in order to determine whether religion truly helps persons to cope or adjust better to stress, we must

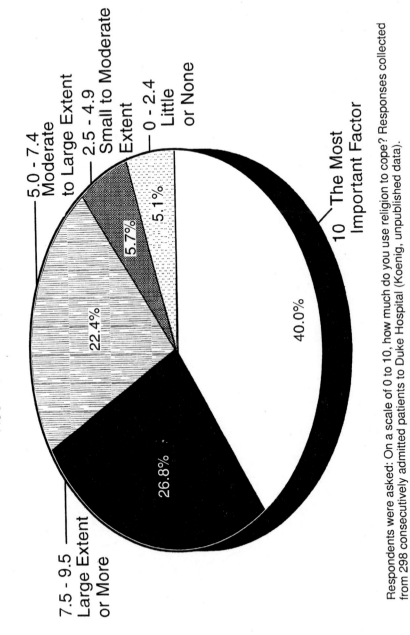

FIGURE 5.1. Self-Related Religious Coping

5.0 - 7.4
Moderate
to Large Extent

2.5 - 4.9
Small to Moderate
Extent

0 - 2.4
Little
or None

10 The Most
Important Factor

7.5 - 9.5
Large Extent
or More

22.4%

5.7%

5.1%

40.0%

26.8%

Respondents were asked: On a scale of 0 to 10, how much do you use religion to cope? Responses collected from 298 consecutively admitted patients to Duke Hospital (Koenig, unpublished data).

FIGURE 5.2. Religious Coping and Severity of Medical Illness

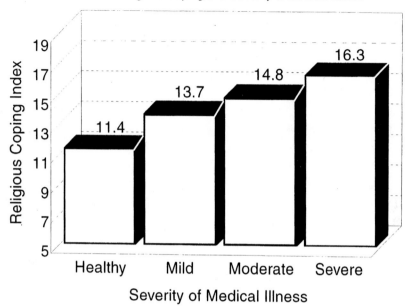

Severity of illness rated by a physician using American Society of Anesthesiologists' illness severity scale.

Source: 1987-1989 Durham, VA, Mental Health Survey of 488 hospitalized patients.

examine whether those who use religion in this way are really more satisfied and happier than those who do not.

## WELL-BEING AND LIFE SATISFACTION

In 1986, our research group examined well-being and religion in a sample of 836 persons over age 60 living in the midwestern United States to determine how religiousness was related to morale and life satisfaction.[7] Standardized self-rated scales were used to measure religiousness (Hoge Intrinsic Religiosity Scale) and morale (Philadelphia Geriatric Center Morale Scale). Participants who frequently attended church, prayed, read the Bible, or were more deeply committed to their faith, experienced significantly higher well-being than those who were less religiously involved (see Figure 5.3). This was true regardless of sex, age, race, physical health, financial status, or level of social support, and was particularly true for women age 75 or older. During a recent conference sponsored by the National Institute on Aging, Andrew Futterman from Holy Cross College and I reported that since 1974 there had been 23 studies of the relationship between religiousness and well-being among older adults. In 21 of these studies, investigators found that persons who were more religious had greater well-being.[8]

FIGURE 5.3. Religion and Well-Being in Older Adults

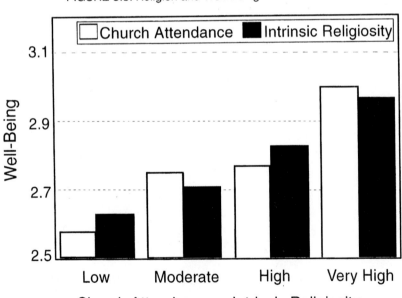

Well-being measured by Philadelphia Geriatric Center Morale Scale.
Religious categories based on quartiles (i.e., low is first quartile, very high is fourth quartile).

Source: Koenig et al. (1988). *The Gerontologist* 28:18-28.

Yes, perhaps religion enhances life satisfaction for older adults. But what about younger persons? Drs. Jeffrey Levin and Christopher Ellison have extensively reviewed the sociological and psychological research on the relationship between religious involvement and well-being among persons of all ages, not just older persons. In addition, they have studied this relationship in their own research involving random samples of persons living throughout the United States. In a series of important scientific papers, these investigators reported positive associations between religious commitment and well-being among persons of all ages, both in their own studies and those of other investigators in the field.[9-12]

These findings, however, have only slowly diffused into medical and psychiatric literature. In general, health professionals are less interested in positive states of mind as they are in *mental disorders* like depression, anxiety, and alcohol or drug abuse—conditions that have a major detrimental effect on health and cause an increase in the use of health services.

## DEPRESSION AND SUICIDE

Most of the adult population of the United States experiences personal or emotional problems at some point or another during the course of a year.[13] About one-half of these people have difficulty solving their problems, and one-third indicate that they cannot do anything to make their problems more bearable. In any given month of the year, about 10 to 15 percent of the population suffers from depression or anxiety severe enough to warrant some form of treatment.[14] Is there a relationship between these emotional problems and religion? Does religion help people to cope better?

Between 1987 and 1989, our research group examined the relationship between the use of religion as a coping behavior and depression in a sample of almost 1,000 hospitalized medically ill men.[6] Patients included in the study were consecutively admitted patients to the medical services of a Veterans Administration hospital in Durham, North Carolina. Depression was measured in several ways. First, patients were asked to rate their own symptoms of feeling sad, blue, disinterested, tired, and so forth. In a subset of 448 patients, a physician rated how severely depressed he thought the patients were. Standard depression scales were used for this purpose (self-rated Geriatric Depression Scale and observer-rated Hamilton Depression Rating Scale).

Religious coping, on the other hand, was measured by three questions. First, patients were asked an open-ended question about what they did that enabled them to cope. Second, patients were asked if they used religion to help them to cope and, if so, to rate how much on a 0 to 10 scale (0 meaning not at all and 10 meaning the most important factor that sustained them). Finally, the interviewers themselves were asked to rate how much they thought the patient used religion as a coping behavior, based on a brief discussion of how religion helped the patient to cope, including examples of what activities they engaged in. This Religious Coping Index was shown to have high inter-rater reliability ($r = 0.81$), even when administered by raters from widely divergent religious backgrounds.

People who used religion as a coping behavior were then compared with those who said they coped in other ways (staying busy, visiting friends or family, and so forth). Patients who depended heavily on their religious faith to cope were significantly less depressed than those who did not (see Figure 5.4). Two hundred and two patients were then followed for an average of six months after they were discharged from the hospital. The objective was to determine what characteristics of patients at study entry would predict who later became depressed. Baseline characteristics of patients included age, marital status, race, financial status, support from family and friends, severity of medical illness, diagnosis, and eight other health and social attributes.

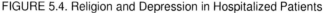

FIGURE 5.4. Religion and Depression in Hospitalized Patients

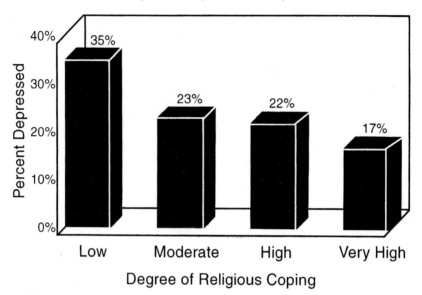

Depression assessed by self-rated Geriatric Depression Scale; religious coping by Religious Coping Index.

Source: Information based on results from 991 consecutively admitted patients (differences significant at p<.0001). Koenig (1994). *Aging and God.* Binghamton, NY: The Haworth Press.

Only two characteristics predicted whether mental health got better or worse. Patients initially diagnosed with severe kidney disease were more likely to be depressed six months after discharge. The only characteristic that predicted lower rates of depression was not the level of support from family or friends, not physical health status, and not even income or education level. Rather, it was the extent to which patients relied on their religious faith to cope. This was the only factor that predicted significantly better mental health six months later (see Figure 5.5). These findings were later published in the *American Journal of Psychiatry*[4] and in *Psychosomatics*.[15]

FIGURE 5.5. Predicators of Change in Depression

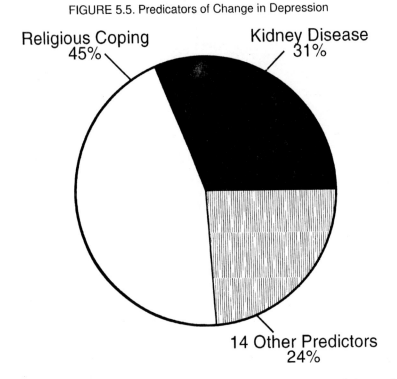

Religious Coping 45%

Kidney Disease 31%

14 Other Predictors 24%

A total of 202 hospitalized patients were followed for an average of six months after discharge. The only significant predicator of lower depression scores was religious coping.

Source: Koenig et al. (1992). *American Journal of Psychiatry* 49:1693-1700.

Also in the late 1980s, our research group conducted a study sponsored by the National Institute on Aging of 4,000 persons in central North Carolina to determine whether those who were more religiously active would be more or less depressed than those who were not religious.[16] Again, persons who attended church at least once a week were only about one-half as likely to be depressed as those who attended church less frequently (the odds ratio was 0.56 with a 95 percent confidence interval of 0.48 to 0.65). The finding was true regardless of age, sex, race, level of social support, and degree of physical illness or functional disability. This study replicated the results obtained in an earlier National Institute of Mental Health (NIMH) study of 2,969 persons of all ages, in which a lower rate of depression was found among frequent church attenders.[17]

These findings contrast with assertions by Dr. Watters in *Deadly Doctrine.* Quoting Kaplan and Sadock's *Textbook of Psychiatry,* Watters notes:[18]

> "It is widely believed that persons prone to depression are characterized by low self-esteem, strong superego, clinging and dependent interpersonal relations, and limited capacity for mature and enduring object relations." As we have demonstrated throughout this book, *these characteristics are inevitable products of the Christian belief system*, one that preaches self-abasement as a means of ingratiating oneself with the deity, that discourages ego growth and inner-directedness, and promotes superego growth and outerdirectedness with its reliance on external authority. (p. 148)

The research team at Duke is not the only research team that has found better adaptation, lower rates of depression, and less frequent negative emotional states among the more religiously active. Investigators in Connecticut,[19,20] Massachusetts,[21] Texas,[22,23] Illinois,[24] California,[25] New York,[26] and other areas of the United States and Canada[8,27,28] have reported similar findings (see Figure 5.6). Included here is the work of Drs. Kennedy, Levin, and Krause, whose research teams have recently examined the relationship between religion and mental health outcomes in a range of populations and locations throughout the country. Gary Kennedy and colleagues in the Department of Psychiatry at Albert Einstein College of Medicine, recently reported that failure to attend church services at least weekly was associated with an almost 40 percent increase in the risk of depression among 1,855 New York City residents.[26]

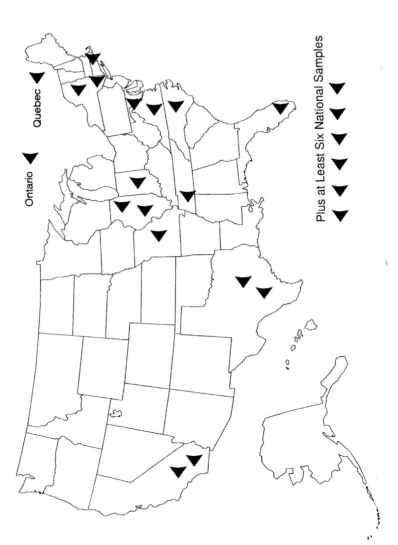

FIGURE 5.6. Locations of a Few of the Studies Showing a Positive Association Between Religion and Mental Health

Quebec

Ontario

Plus at Least Six National Samples

Examining a national sample of black Americans, Jeffrey Levin and colleagues found that persons who were more religiously involved experienced significantly greater life satisfaction, even after taking into account the effects of physical health status and other conventional predictors of well-being.[29] This is one of the most methodologically advanced studies to date because it takes advantage of the latest advances in statistical analysis (structural equation modeling). Levin's research team also recently reported results from a study of 624 Mexican Americans from Texas who had been followed for over a decade. These investigators found that frequency of church attendance among the *youngest* members in their study (mean age 27) predicted lower depression and more positive attitudes toward life 11 years later.[30]

Self-esteem is another important mental health outcome because a lack of it has been strongly linked with depression. Dr. Watters spends almost five pages in *Deadly Doctrine* (pp. 50-54) describing the allegedly negative effects of Christian teachings on self-esteem. Krause and colleagues at the School of Public Health, University of Michigan, have recently put Dr. Watters' opinions to the test. They examined the relationship between religious coping and self-esteem in a large, predominantly Christian sample, and found that persons who relied heavily on religion to cope actually had very high levels of self-esteem. They concluded that feelings of self-worth "tend to be lowest for those with very little religious commitment" (p. 236).[31]

Consistent with the findings of higher self-esteem and lower depression among religiously active persons, a number of researchers have now reported lower rates of suicide (the most dire consequence of depression) among those who are more religiously involved[32-35] (see Figure 5.7). Again, this is the opposite of what some mental health experts would have predicted. The claim that these findings are due, as Watters contends (pp. 153-157), to "social desirability" of subjects' responses or the tendency for religious persons to "deny emergency emotions," is weak when

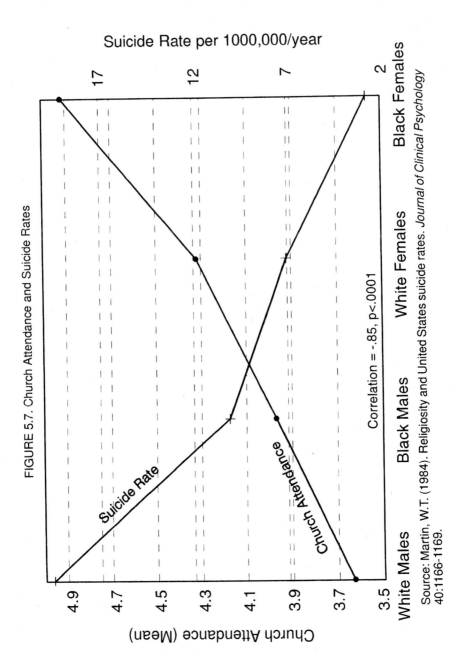

FIGURE 5.7. Church Attendance and Suicide Rates

Suicide Rate per 1000,000/year

Church Attendance (Mean)

Suicide Rate

Church Attendance

Correlation = -.85, p<.0001

White Males    Black Males    White Females    Black Females

Source: Martin, W.T. (1984). Religiosity and United States suicide rates. *Journal of Clinical Psychology* 40:1166-1169.

one considers that these findings were made by different research teams, working in different areas of the country, at different points in time.

## *ANXIETY*

Like depression, anxiety and worry are widespread in America today. This is true despite the fact that there is perhaps less reason to feel anxious in this country than in almost any other place in the world (given the relative absence of war, severe poverty, and political instability which characterize many other countries). Indeed, tranquilizers, antihypertensives, and anti-ulcer drugs are the most commonly prescribed drugs by physicians in the United States. Religious beliefs also promise relief from anxiety, stress, and worry, though it is possible that they might also increase anxiety by arousing guilt over sins and worry about divine retribution.

In the early 1980s our research team conducted a study sponsored by the NIMH to examine the relationship between anxiety and religious activity in a sample of almost 3,000 persons living in North Carolina. It was found that frequent church attenders actually experienced significantly lower rates of anxiety disorder than did infrequent attenders and those with no religious affiliation.[36] These results were strongest among *younger* persons ages 18 to 39 (in other words, baby boomers) (see Figure 5.8). Other investigators have reported similar results (lower levels of anxiety among the more religious) in samples of both healthy and medically ill subjects.[37-39]

## *ALCOHOL AND DRUG ABUSE*

Alcohol and drug abuse are among the most serious problems that plague society today. They cause serious health problems

FIGURE 5.8. Church Attendance and Anxiety Disorder

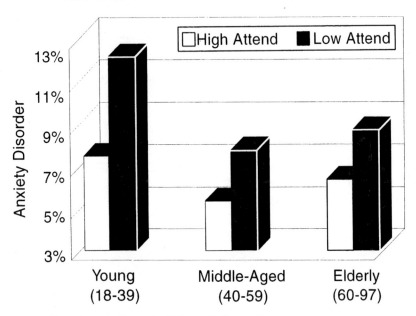

Anxiety disorder experienced within past six months.

Source: Epidemiologic Catchment Area survey (1983-1984), North Carolina site, of 2,964 community-dwelling adults. Koenig et al. (1993). *Journal of Anxiety Disorders* 7:321-342.

and driving accidents, they destroy families and ruin young people's futures, and they are strongly associated with criminal activity and imprisonment. Alcohol is at least partly responsible for almost one-half of all deaths caused by motor vehicle crashes, suicides, and homicides.[40] In 1983, alcohol problems in America exceeded $70 billion per year, and drug problems accounted for $44 billion per year.[41] The cost to society, then, both in economic terms and in human life, is enormous. Any resource that might reduce alcohol or drug abuse even a small amount could yield immense benefits to society.

Most religions discourage excess use of alcohol and other substances that harm the body. In an NIMH-sponsored study of several thousand persons of all ages, our research group examined the relationship between alcoholism and religious activities was examined.[42] Persons who frequently attended church (at least once a week), prayed or read the Bible, or considered themselves "born again" had significantly lower rates of alcoholism. In fact, frequent church attenders were less than one-third as likely (odds ratio 0.29) as less frequent attenders were to experience alcoholism within six months prior to the survey and were less than one-half as likely (odds ratio 0.48) to ever have the diagnosis (see Figure 5.9). This study adds to the growing body of literature that shows a connection between religiousness and low rates of alcohol and drug use among people of all ages.[43-50]

FIGURE 5.9. Church Attendance and Alcoholism

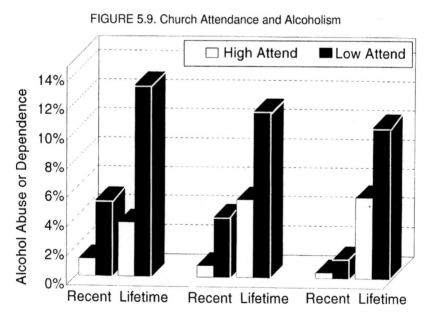

Recent = within past six months.

Source: NIMH Epidemiologic Catchment Area Survey (1983-1984), North Carolina site, of 2,964 participants of all ages. Koenig et al. (1994). *Hospital and Community Psychiatry* 45:225-231.

Almost every study that has ever examined the relationship between religion and substance abuse has found lower rates of abuse among the more religious. Besides the existence of religious doctrines that discourage excess alcohol or drug use, religious communities help prevent addictions (or facilitate recovery) through community support, individual commitment, and belief in a higher power—many of the same principles that operate therapeutically in Alcoholics Anonymous. According to Harvard professor George Vaillant,[51]

> . . . alcoholics and victims of other seemingly incurable habits feel defeated, bad, and helpless. They invariably suffer from impaired morale. If they are to recover, powerful new sources of self-esteem and hope must be discovered. Religion is one such source. Religion provides fresh impetus for both hope and enhanced self-care. Second, if the established alcoholic is to become stably abstinent, enormous personality changes must take place. It is not just coincidence that we associated such dramatic change with the experience of religious conversion. Third, religion, in ways that we appreciate but do not understand, provides forgiveness of sins and relief from guilt. Unlike many intractable habits that others find merely annoying, alcoholism inflicts enormous pain and injury on those around the alcoholic. As a result the alcoholic, already demoralized by his inability to stop drinking, experiences almost insurmountable guilt from the torture he has inflicted on others. In such an instance, absolution becomes an important part of the healing process. (p. 193)

## TREATMENT STUDIES

Some of the most powerful evidence for religion's positive effects on mental health comes from studies that have successfully used religious interventions to treat emotional disorders. Propst and colleagues[52] in Oregon compared the effectiveness of two types of cognitive-behavioral psychotherapy (CBT) in the treatment of depressed patients (average age 40 years). One version was a standard treatment protocol (secular CBT); the other version included religious content based on counseling practices used by Protestant and Catholic clergy (religious CBT). Religious CBT gave Christian rationales for restructuring thought processes, used religious arguments to counter irrational thoughts, and used religious imagery as part of the behavioral component. Forty religious patients were randomly assigned to either secular CBT, religious CBT, a pastoral counseling group, or a control group that received no treatment. Results showed that religious CBT and pastoral counseling groups responded much quicker (by reduced depression) than did either secular CBT or control groups.

A second study assessed the effectiveness of religious interventions in the treatment of Muslim patients with anxiety disorder.[53] Sixty-two patients (average age 40 years) were randomly assigned to treatment or control groups. Both groups received medication and supportive psychotherapy for anxiety. In addition, however, one group received a religious intervention that involved prayer and having patients read verses from the Holy Koran. After three months, the religious intervention group scored significantly lower on anxiety tests than did the group without religious treatment.

## POSSIBLE MECHANISMS OF EFFECT

There are at least three natural mechanisms by which religion might promote mental health: first, through a system of beliefs and mental attitudes; second, through increased social support and promotion of interaction with others; and third, by emphasizing a focus on others and on a power higher than the self. I will use Christian beliefs to illustrate these mechanisms, although other belief systems may operate in a similar manner.

First, religious beliefs provide hope and a sense of control over one's destiny. Judeo-Christian scriptures emphasize that something good can result from every situation if the believer puts his or her complete trust in God. God is depicted as a personal God who is involved and interested in creation, especially in humans who were created in the Creator's image and are more like God than is anything else in creation. God is portrayed as caring about every individual in a personal way and wanting to be involved in their life. This is a God who can be reached and influenced by personal prayer and who actually desires such communication.

In this belief system, anyone can at any time and in any place talk with the all-powerful, all-present, all-knowing, all-merciful Creator and Sustainer of the universe, and can influence what God does; and if not influence what God does, then receive strength to cope with whatever adversity may come along. Even death itself is no victor over the believer whose soul is immortal. There is no sin or mistake in life that cannot be confessed and forgiven. Thus, no matter what a person has done in the past, he or she can start life fresh again by recommitting one's life to God. Guilt, which religion itself can provoke, is erased by the simple act of asking for forgiveness. Not surprisingly, such beliefs may have powerful psychological consequences, and may indeed bring comfort to those who are lonely, anxious, discouraged, or feeling out of control.

Second, active participation in the religious community brings people into contact with others of similar age who have common interests and with whom social relationships may form. Religious doctrines promote social interaction by encouraging positive social attitudes and self-sacrifice ("love thy neighbor"). Studies have shown that church attendance is strongly related to almost every dimension of social support.[54] For those in certain age groups–especially the elderly–support from church members exceeds that from all other sources combined (other than family members).[55] Social support, in turn, is related to lower rates of depression, anxiety, loneliness, and other mental health problems.[56] Indeed, emotional support from others is a major therapeutic tool used in all forms of counseling and psychotherapy.

Religion's social effects include its impact on the family unit and on the rearing of children. Studies have shown that religiously active marriages are more satisfying and less prone to divorce.[57-62] Intact family units are available to provide emotional support and care for members when they become sick or face tragedy. Religious families are also likely to instill religious values in children, stressing commitment and character development, including honor and respect for parents. These values may later affect whether children are willing to help out aging parents or siblings. The future care of older adults in society may rest on such values.

Third, religious doctrines promote a healthy, balanced love of God, self, and others. As noted earlier, most persons in today's society strive for independence, self-sufficiency, and self-promotion, rather than seeking to help or improve the lot of others. This trend is reinforced by pop psychology, which focuses on self-help, self-development, self-fulfillment, and so forth. The message sent by Judeo-Christian beliefs is quite different: stop focusing on yourself, and start focusing on God; serve God, not yourself; the surest path to self-fulfillment, happiness, and self-esteem is not through striving to achieve these things for the self, but rather through providing these to others because of love for God and desire to serve God.

Obedience, service, self-sacrifice, bearing other's burdens–these are things we run away from in today's world; to the contrary, Christianity and Judaism say to embrace them, practice them, and devote one's life to them. Indeed, many emotional disorders today result from people being focused on or preoccupied with their own petty issues. Religion says that a cure for such narcissistic tendencies is to transcend the self, put trust in a power higher than the self, and be concerned with loving and helping others. Again, these are the same principles by which Alcoholics Anonymous and many drug-recovery programs operate; their overwhelming success when compared with many secular rehabilitation programs testifies to their effectiveness. These attitudes are also the very fabric which holds families, communities, and nations together.

### Generalizing Across Religious Groups

Do all religions have the same effect? It is difficult to say. Systematic research that has examined the associations between religion and mental health has been conducted primarily in countries where the Judeo-Christian religion predominates. At this time, then, one can safely apply conclusions only to persons with this particular religious background. There is limited research that suggests the results may apply to other faith traditions as well[53,63]; nevertheless, the number of these studies is quite small and further research is clearly needed. The content of religious belief—*what* people believe—appears to be quite important in the mechanism by which religion conveys its positive effects on mental health (see above). Because the content of belief differs between different religions, the effects on mental health may differ as well.

### Generalizing to Spirituality

Can these findings be applied to "spirituality" in general? Again, it is difficult to say. "Spirituality" is a much more acceptable term than religion and has achieved great popularity in today's culture. The mental health benefits of traditional religious beliefs and practices, however, may or may not apply to spirituality. While spirituality includes traditional religious belief and practice, it is a much broader term that extends far beyond, to include New Age forms of spirituality, parapsychology (telepathy, extrasensory perception, clairvoyance, other psychic phenomena), and astrology. Almost every known human and mystical experience has been included under this term. Consequently, researchers have not been able to agree on a universal definition that can be operationalized and measured. This makes spirituality, apart from traditional religious belief and practice, difficult to study. Indeed, the vast majority of research today that talks about spirituality and its effects on health, in reality, examines only religion.[63] Research that measures spirituality (separate from religious belief, practice, or commitment) needs to be done in order to see if the health benefits of religion generalize to this broader concept.

## *SUMMARY*

Is religion good for your mental health? Let's summarize the evidence. First, when persons are asked an open-ended question about what enables them to cope with stress, they frequently say that religion (faith in God, prayer, scripture reading, church) comforts and brings relief from anxiety and despair. Second, when persons are studied, using the standard research methodology, those who are more religious are less depressed, anxious, and cope better with adversity. Third, we can predict ahead of time who will and will not become depressed based, at least in part, on whether or not persons use religion as a coping behavior. Fourth, when religion is integrated into traditional treatments for depression and anxiety, better results are achieved than those obtained by standard secular approaches alone (especially in religious patients). These research findings argue against Freud's and other health professionals' assertions that religion has a negative or neurotic influence on mental health. Indeed, the opposite appears to be true. There are three natural mechanisms by which religious belief and practice may promote mental health, and these are reviewed. We do not yet know whether all religions have the same effect in this regard, or if the findings can be generalized to the broader concept of "spirituality."

## REFERENCE NOTES

1. Princeton Religion Research Center. (1982). *Religion in America*. Princeton, NJ: Gallup Poll.

2. Americana Healthcare Corporation. (1980-1981). *Aging in America: Trials and Triumphs*. Westport, CT: Survey Sampling (for Research & Forecasts, Inc).

3. Koenig, H.G., L.K. George, and I. Siegler. (1988). The use of religion and other emotion-regulating coping strategies among older adults. *The Gerontologist* 28:303-310.

4. Koenig, H.G., H.J. Cohen, D.G. Blazer, C. Pieper, K.G. Meador, F. Shelp, V. Goli, R. DiPasquale. (1992). Religious coping and depression in elderly hospitalized medically ill men. *American Journal of Psychiatry* 149:1693-1700.

5. Koenig, H.G. (1996). Depressive disorder in hospitalized medically ill elders (unpublished data). Funded by National Institutes of Mental Health, grant # MH01138. (1993-1998).

6. Koenig, H.G. (1994). *Aging and God*. Binghamton, NY: The Haworth Press.

7. Koenig, H.G., J.N. Kvale, and C. Ferrel. (1988). Religion and well-being in later life. *The Gerontologist* 28:18-28.

8. Koenig, H.G., and A. Futterman. (1995). Religion and health outcomes: A review and synthesis of the literature. Background paper, published in proceedings of *Conference on Methodological Approaches to the Study of Religion, Aging, and Health*. Sponsored by the National Institute on Aging. (March 16-17, 1996.)

9. Levin, J.S., and K.S. Markides. (1988). Religious attendance and psychological well-being in middle-aged and older Mexican Americans. *Sociological Analysis* 49:66-72.

10. Levin, J.S., L.M. Chatters, and R.J. Taylor. (1994). Religious effects on health status and life satisfaction among Black Americans. *Journal of Gerontology*. (Social Sciences) 50B:S154-S163.

11. Ellison, C.G., D.A. Gay, and T.A. Glass. (1989). Does religious commitment contribute to individual life satisfaction? *Social Forces* 68:100-123.

12. Ellison, C.G. (1991). Religious involvement and subjective well-being. *Journal of Health and Social Behavior* 32:80-99.

13. *Healthy People 2000*. (1991). National Health Promotion and Disease Prevention: U.S. Department of Health and Human Services, Public Health Service, DHHS Publication No. (PHS) 91-50212.

14. Regier, D.A., J.H. Boyd, J.D. Burke, D.S. Rae, J.K. Myers, M. Kramer, L.N. Robins, L.K. George, M. Karno, and B.Z. Locke. (1988). One-month preva-

lence of mental disorders in the United States. *Archives of General Psychiatry* 45:977-986.

15. Koenig, H.G., H.J. Cohen, D.G. Blazer, and K.R.R. Krishnan. (1995). Religious coping and cognitive symptoms of depression in elderly medical patients. *Psychosomatics* 36:369-375.

16. Koenig, H.G., J.C. Hays, L.K. George, and D.G. Blazer. (1996). Modeling the impact of chronic illness, religion, and social support on depressive symptoms. Paper presented at the *American Association for the Advancement of Science* annual meeting, Baltimore, Maryland, February 11, 1996.

17. Koenig, H.G., L.K. George, K.G. Meador, D.G. Blazer, and P.B. Dyck. (1994). Religious affiliation and psychiatric disorder among Protestant baby boomers. *Hospital & Community Psychiatry* 45:586-596.

18. Watters, Wendell W., MD. (1992). *Deadly Doctrine: Health, Illness, and Christian God-Talk*. Amherst, NY: Prometheus Books. Reprinted by permission of the publisher.

19. Idler, E.L. (1987). Religious involvement and the health of the elderly. *Social Forces* 66:226-238.

20. Idler, E.L., and S.V. Kasl. (1992). Religion, disability, depression, and the timing of death. *American Journal of Sociology* 97:1052-1079.

21. Morse, C.K., and P.A. Wisocki. (1987). Importance of religiosity to elderly adjustment. *Journal of Religion and Aging* 4(1):15-28.

22. Nelson, P.B. (1989). Ethnic differences in intrinsic/extrinsic religious orientation and depression in the elderly. *Archives of Psychiatric Nursing* 3(4):199-204.

23. Nelson, P.B. (1989). Social support, self-esteem, and depression in the institutionalized elderly. *Issues in Mental Health Nursing* 10:55-68.

24. Pressman, P., J.S. Lyons, D.B. Larson, and J.S. Strain. (1990). Religious belief, depression, and ambulation status in elderly women with broken hips. *American Journal of Psychiatry* 147:758-760.

25. Nelson, F.L. (1977). Religiosity and self-destructive crises in the institutionalized elderly. *Suicide and Life-Threatening Behavior* 7:67-74.

26. Kennedy, G.J., H.R. Kelman, C. Thomas, and J. Chen. (1996). Religious affiliation, practice and depression among 1,855 older community residents. *Journal of Gerontology* (Psychological Sciences), in press.

27. O'Connor, B.P., and R.J. Vallerand. (1990). Religious motivation in the elderly. A French-Canadian replication and an extension. *Journal of Social Psychology* 130:53-59.

28. Matthews, D.A., and D.B. Larson. (1993-1996). *The Faith Factor: An Annotated Bibliography of Clinical Research on Spiritual Subjects*. Vols. I-IV. Rockville, MD: National Institute for Healthcare Research.

29. Levin, J.S., L.M. Chatters, and R.J. Taylor. (1995). Religious effects on health status and life satisfaction among black Americans. *Journal of Gerontology* (Social Sciences) 50B:S154-S163.

30. Levin, J.S., K.S. Markides, and L.A. Ray. (1996). Religious attendance and psychological well-being in Mexican Americans: A panel analysis of three-generations data. *The Gerontologist*, in press.

31. Krause, N. (1995). Religiosity and self-esteem among older adults. *Journal of Gerontology* (Psychological Sciences) 50:P236-P246.

32. Martin, W.T. (1984). Religiosity and United States suicide rates, 1972-1978. *Journal of Clinical Psychology* 40(5):1166-1169.

33. Stack, S. (1983). The effect of religious commitment on suicide: A cross-national analysis. *Journal of Health and Social Behavior*, (pp. 362-374).

34. Stack, S. (1983). The effect of religiosity on suicide. *Journal for the Scientific Study of Religion*, 22:239-252.

35. Breault, K.D., and K. Barkey. (1982). A comparative analysis of Durkheim's theory of egoistic suicide. *The Sociological Quarterly* 23:321-331.

36. Koenig, H.G., S.M. Ford, L.K. George, D.G. Blazer, K.G. Meador. (1993). Religion and anxiety disorder: An examination and comparison of associations in young, middle-aged, and elderly adults. *Journal of Anxiety Disorders* 7:321-342.

37. Thorson, J.A., and F.C. Powell. (1990). Meanings of death and intrinsic religiosity. *Journal of Clinical Psychology* 46:379-391.

38. Kaczorowski, J.M. (1989). Spiritual well-being and anxiety in adults diagnosed with cancer. *The Hospice Journal* 5(3/4):105-116.

39. Morris, P.A. (1982). The effect of pilgrimage on anxiety, depression, and religious attitudes. *Psychological Medicine* 12:291-294.

40. Perrine, M., R. Peck, and J. Fell. (1989). Epidemiologic perspectives on drunk driving. *Surgeon General's Workshop on Drunk Driving: Background Papers*. Washington, DC: U.S. Department of Health and Human Services.

41. Rice, D.P., L.S. Kelman, and S. Dunmeyer. (1990). *The Economic Costs of Alcohol and Drug Abuse and Mental Illness*. San Francisco, CA: Institute for Health and Aging, University of California at San Francisco.

42. Koenig, H.G., L.K. George, K.G. Meador, D.G. Blazer, and S.M. Ford. (1994). Religious practices and alcoholism in a southern adult population. *Hospital & Community Psychiatry* 45:225-237.

43. Parfrey, P.S. (1976). The effect of religious factors on intoxicant use. *Scandinavian Journal of Social Medicine* 3:135-140.

44. Larson, D.B., and W.P. Wilson. (1980). Religious life of alcoholics. *Southern Medical Journal* 73:723-727.

45. Khavari, K.A., and T.M. Harmon. (1982). The relationship between degree of professed religious belief and use of drugs. *International Journal of Addictions* 17:847-857.

46. Coombs, R.H., D.K. Wellisch, and F.I. Fawzy. (1985). Drinking patterns and problems among female children and adolescents: A comparison of abstainers, past users, and current users. *American Journal of Drug and Alcohol Abuse* 11:315-348.

47. Hilton, M.E. (1991). The demographic distribution of drinking problems in 1984. In W.B. Clark and M.E. Hilton (Eds.), *Alcohol in America: Drinking Practices and Problems* (pp. 87-101).

48. Beeghley, L., E.W. Bock, and J.K. Cochran. (1990). Religious change and alcohol use: An application of reference group and socialization theory. *Sociological Forum* 5:261-278.

49. Krause, N. (1991). Stress, religiosity, and abstinence from alcohol. *Psychology and Aging* 6:134-144.

50. Alexander, F., and R.W. Duff. (1991). Influence of religiosity and alcohol use on personal well-being. *Journal of Religious Gerontology* 8(2):11-21.

51. Vaillant, G.E. (1983). Paths into abstinence. In G.E. Vaillant (Ed.) *The Natural History of Alcoholism: Causes, Patterns and Paths to Recovery.* Cambridge, MA: Harvard University Press, pp. 193-194.

52. Propst, L.R., R. Ostrom, P. Watkins, T. Dean, and D. Mashburn. (1992). Comparative efficacy of religious and nonreligious cognitive-behavioral therapy for the treatment of clinical depression in religious individuals. *Journal of Consulting and Clinical Psychology* 60:94-103.

53. Azhart, M.A., S.L. Varma, and A.S. Dharap. (1994). Religious psychotherapy in anxiety disorder patients. *Acta Psychiatrica Scandinavica* 90:1-3.

54. Ellison, C.G., and L.K. George. (1994). Religious involvement, social ties, and social support in a Southeastern community. *Journal for the Scientific Study of Religion* 33:46-61.

55. Koenig, H.G., D.O. Moberg, and J.N. Kvale. (1988). Religious activities and attitudes of older adults in a geriatric assessment clinic. *Journal of the American Geriatrics Society* 36:362-374.

56. George, L.K. (1995). Social and economic factors related to psychiatric disorders in late life. In E.W. Busse and D.G. Blazer (Eds.) *Geriatric Psychiatry* (2nd edition). Washington, DC: American Psychiatric Press.

57. Wilson, M.R., and E.E. Filsinger. (1986). Religiosity and marital adjustment: multidimensional interrelationships. *Journal of Marriage and the Family* 48:147-151.

58. Dudley, M.G., and F.A. Kosinski. (1990). Religiosity and marital satisfaction: a research note. *Review of Religious Research* 32:78-86.

59. Schumm, W.R., S.R. Bollman, and A.P. Jurich. (1982). The "marital conventionalization" argument: Implications for the study of religiosity and marital satisfaction. *Journal of Psychology and Theology* 10:236-241.

60. Robinson, L.C. (1994). Religious orientation in enduring marriage: an exploratory study. *Review of Religious Research* 35:207-218.

61. Sporakowski, M.J., and G.A. Hughston. (1978). Prescriptions for happy marriage: adjustments and satisfactions of couples married for 50 or more years. *The Family Coordinator* 321-327.

62. Roth, P.D. (1988). Spiritual well-being and marital adjustment. *Journal of Psychology and Theology* 16:153-158.

63. Shams, M., and P.R. Jackson. (1993). Religiosity as a predictor of well-being and moderator of the psychological impact of unemployment. *Journal of Medical Psychology* 66:341-352.

64. Levin, J.S. (1996). How religion influences morbidity and health: Reflections on natural history, salutogenesis, and host resistance. *Social Science and Medicine,* in press.

# Chapter 6

# Religion and Physical Health

When the question "Is religion good for your health?" comes up, most of us are particularly interested in religion's effects on *physical health*. If the religiously involved person is more satisfied with life, less depressed, and less anxious, do these positive effects on mental health also translate into better physical health and longer life? When I first began searching medical literature for studies on religion and mental health, I could locate only a few studies. Just about that time, Dr. Jeffrey Levin was doing an exhaustive search of the broader topic of religion and physical health. He found over 200 studies that had examined some aspect of this topic. Dr. Levin had a difficult time getting his paper published because of the negative and sometimes degrading attitude of medical journal editors. He finally published it in a pastoral care journal that most medical and psychiatric researchers do not read,[1] and so this information remained hidden for some time. The vast majority of studies Dr. Levin referred to in his review examined associations between religious *affiliation* and different physical illnesses. Associations were usually explained on the basis of diet or other health practices. Little attention, however, was paid by researchers in these studies to the effects of *religiousness per se* (our primary interest here) on health.

Over the past ten years, however, a number of well-designed studies published in reputable medical journals have found a relationship between religiousness and lower rates of specific physical diseases, as well as lower overall mortality[2] (see Figure

6.1). I will review some of these studies here. Before proceeding, however, it will be helpful to present a theoretical model that explains *why* strong religious commitment and devout religious practice might result in better physical health[3] (see Figure 6.2). This model can be used to understand and interpret the findings I present in the rest of this chapter.

## *DIRECT AND INDIRECT INFLUENCES*

Religiousness can affect health directly by two major mechanisms, and indirectly by two others. None of these mechanisms

FIGURE 6.1. The Relationship Between Religion and Mortality

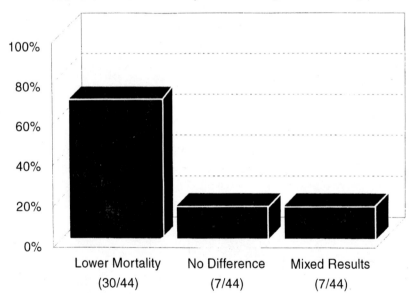

| Lower Mortality | No Difference | Mixed Results |
| (30/44) | (7/44) | (7/44) |

Based on a systematic review of the literature from 1933-1995. Forty-four studies are identified that statistically examined the relationship between religion and mortality.

Source: Larson and Koenig (1996). Does religion prolong your life? (unpublished manuscript) Supported by the John Templeton Foundation.

FIGURE 6.2. Prevention Model for Religion's Effects on Physical Health

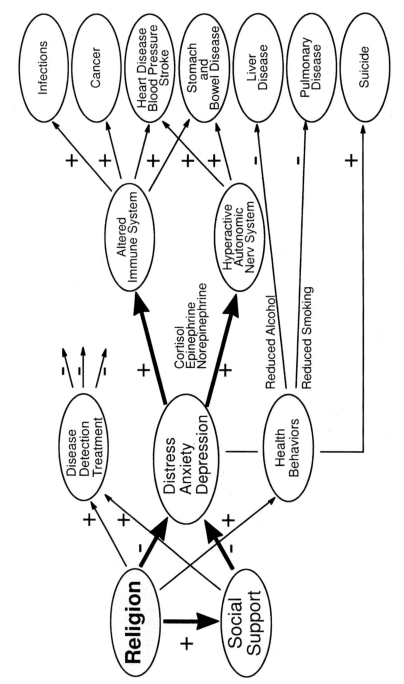

involve "supernatural," "superempirical," or "nonlocal" effects, but rather can be explained by known naturalistic physiological pathways. The two *direct* mechanisms involve (1) earlier diagnosis and better treatment of physical diseases, and (2) reduction in behaviors that adversely affect health (decreased smoking, drinking, unsafe sexual practices, diet, and so forth). The two *indirect* mechanisms involve (1) an enhancement of social support, and (2) a reduction of distress, depression, anxiety, and other emotional disorders.

### Direct Effects

Among the direct pathways by which religion might improve health and prolong survival is by promoting early disease detection and ensuring adequate treatment. Religious teachings emphasize respect for one's physical body. Religious individuals may pay closer attention to their physical health because, according to Christian teachings, their bodies are "temples of the Holy Spirit." Religious persons may also be more compliant and likely to follow medical treatment regimens more scrupulously.[4] As mentioned earlier, religiously active persons have broader social support systems that may encourage them to seek treatment early for health problems, take them to the doctor, and remind them to comply with treatment that is ordered.

The second direct pathway by which religious commitment might affect health is by discouraging behaviors such as excess alcohol and drug use, smoking, risky sexual behaviors, and several other activities that adversely affect health. In the last chapter, we showed how alcohol and drug abuse or dependence are much lower among those who are religiously active. Likewise, lower rates of cigarette smoking have been documented in the religiously involved.[5] The positive health effects of low-risk lifestyles and healthy diet are most evident among religious groups like Mormons and Seventh-Day Adventists, who have lower mortality from cancer, heart disease, and other diseases, than do members of the general population.[2]

### Indirect Effects

An indirect way that religion might influence health is through its link with social support. As noted in the last chapter, a number of studies have now documented a strong association between religious activity and support from others. Involvement in a religious community enhances supportive relationships, which benefit health because they provide a sense of belonging,[6-8] give people a reason for living that transcends themselves,[9] and in a variety of ways influence people to practice more preventative and therapeutically healthy behaviors.[9,10] Social behaviors may also enhance a person's "sense of coherence" and thus, their will to live.[8] Recent research seems to bear this out. A relationship between high levels of social support and survival has been repeatedly demonstrated both epidemiologically[11-14] and in clinical trials.[15]

Among the clinical trials is a study by David Spiegel and colleagues[15] at Stanford University. These investigators assigned 86 patients with metastatic breast cancer to either a control group which received routine cancer care (n = 36) or to an intervention group which received 12 months of weekly supportive group therapy (n = 50). Survival times between the two groups were compared at ten years. Patients receiving supportive group therapy survived nearly twice as long as those in the control group (36.6 months vs. 18.9 months). This study provides solid rationale for how religion, by surrounding the individual with a supportive, nurturing community, might enhance survival.

A second indirect effect of religion on health, one which may be the most important yet, is its effects on mental health. As noted in the previous chapter, a link between religiousness, social support, and mental health has been documented in a number of studies. Not only might this explanation result in lower rates of mortality from suicide,[16-19] but also from the devastating physiological effects that chronic stress and depression have on the body. Persons who are depressed have increased secretion of cortisol from their adrenal glands. This natural substance interferes with the immune system,[20-25] which is the body's major defense against cancer,[26,27] infections, and other outside invaders. In fact, this is the substance that doctors give patients who receive heart, kidney, or liver transplants to suppress their immune system so that their bodies will not reject the transplanted organ.

Psychological distress also causes the adrenal glands to secrete epinephrine and norepinephrine—substances that cause constriction of blood vessels, which may contribute to high blood pressure, diseases of the arteries that feed the heart (coronary arteries), and possibly irregularities in heart rhythm (arrhythmias).[28-30] Finally, psychological stress increases activity in a part of the nervous system called the autonomic nervous system, which may cause or worsen heart and blood vessel problems, as well as induce stomach ulcers,[31] and may lower bowel or colon problems (irritable bowel syndrome).[32] Consequently, persons with emotional problems such as depression, anxiety, or those who are under chronic stress, may be at greater risk of dying from a number of stress-related diseases.[33,34]

There are multiple pathways, then, by which religious commitment, together with strong social support, may positively influence health and ultimately affect survival. Let us now review research that has examined the relationship between religion and specific physical health conditions.

## DISEASES OF THE BLOOD VESSELS AND HEART

I have already discussed the physiological changes that psychological stress triggers, and the negative effects these can have on the heart and blood vessels of the body. In addition, we know that certain health behaviors like smoking and use of alcohol affect the cardiovascular system. In this section, I will look at the relationship between religious behaviors and three physical conditions: high blood pressure, heart disease, and stroke.

### High Blood Pressure

Between 20 and 30 percent of adults in America have high blood pressure (a blood pressure above 140 mm Hg systolic and/or 90 mm Hg diastolic and/or taking antihypertensive medication).[35] For black Americans, the figure reaches as high as 40 percent. High blood pressure adversely affects the heart, the kidneys, and the brain. Persons with high blood pressure are at greater risk for heart attack, heart failure, kidney failure, and especially stroke. While high blood pressure has strong hereditary and biological components, a number of studies have now linked high blood pressure with anxiety, repressed hostility, and psychological stress.[36-40]

The effects of both church attendance and the importance of religion on blood pressures were examined in 407 men (all ages) who participated in the Evans County, Georgia, Cardiovascular Study.[41] It was found that men who either attended church frequently (once a week or more) or reported that religion was very important to them, had lower systolic and lower diastolic blood pressures than did men who were not religiously involved. The effect was greatest in those who both attended church frequently *and* reported that religion was very important to them; these men had average diastolic blood pressures that were five points lower than those in the low frequency, low importance group (see Figure 6.3). This difference in blood pressure is clinically important, and could mean the difference between a person needing treatment or not.

At least eight other studies have now examined the relationship between religion and blood pressure.[42-49] Seven of these eight studies also reported lower blood pressures for those who were more religiously active. Differences in both systolic and

FIGURE 6.3. Effects of Religiousness on Diastolic Blood Pressure

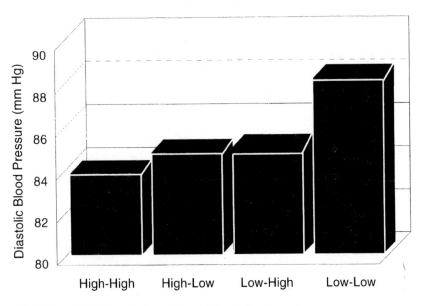

High-High: high church attendance, high religion importance.
Low-Low: low church attendance, low religion importance.

Source: Data from 407 men in the Evans County Cardiovascular Epidemiologic Study (p<.005). Larson, D., H. Koenig, B. Kaplan et al. (1989). *Journal of Religion and Health* 28:265-278.

diastolic blood pressures were found. Of studies that actually measured blood pressures and took into account other factors that might affect blood pressure (weight, age, sex, and so forth), all found lower blood pressures among the more religious.

### *Stroke*

Among the most dreaded complications of high blood pressure is stroke. Every 1.2 minutes, someone in the United States becomes a victim of stroke, the third most common cause of death in this country. Among whites, more than 30 per 100,000 persons in this country die each year from stroke; among blacks, the rate is over

50 per 100,000.[50] In addition, nearly 500,000 persons experience a nonfatal stroke each year in the United States, most of whom remain disabled. It has been estimated that the cost of care plus loss of earnings due to stroke is well over 10 billion dollars per year in the United States.[51]

To my knowledge, there has been only one study that has directly examined the relationship between religiousness and stroke.[52] Investigators from Yale University looked at the rate of new stroke during a six-year period among 2,812 persons age 65 or over living in Connecticut. They examined three religious factors: frequency of attendance at religious services, self-rated religiosity, and religion as a source of strength. Investigators found lower rates of stroke in persons who attended religious services at least once per week and in those who reported a great deal of comfort from religion. The largest difference was for church attendance. Those who never or almost never attended church had nearly double the rate of stroke as did those who attended church on a weekly or more frequent basis. Note, however, that persons who attended church irregularly (a couple of times a month) had the highest risk (see Figure 6.4).

### Heart Disease

Heart disease is by far the most common cause of death for both men and women in the United States. Most heart problems result from diseases of the coronary arteries (vessels that provide blood to the heart), heart valves, or heart rhythm. Coronary heart disease alone affects about 7 million Americans and kills more than 500,000 persons each year.[53] As noted earlier, psychological and social factors are known to affect the heart. Indeed, "the heart" is often used synonymously with emotions (for example, "She broke my heart"). A number of studies have now examined the relationship between religious commitment and heart disease.

FIGURE 6.4. Church Attendance and Stroke (Likelihood of stroke over six years)

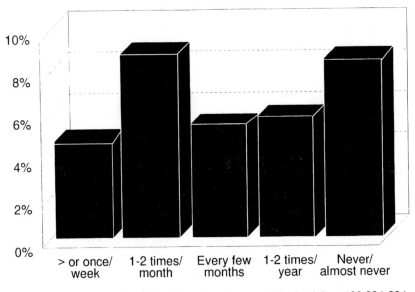

Source: Colantonio et al. (1992). *American Journal of Epidemiology* 136:884-894.

In 1963, Wardwell and colleagues first reported evidence for an association between heart disease and religiousness, finding that heart attacks were less common among persons born from a religiously homogenous marriage (both parents with the same religious affiliation).[54] It was almost a decade later that epidemiologist George Comstock at Johns Hopkins University noted a relationship between coronary artery disease and frequency of church attendance. In the study, infrequent church attenders experienced nearly twice the risk of death from atherosclerotic cardiovascular disease as did frequent church attenders.[55,56] At about this time, Jack Medalie from Case Western Reserve University was examining the association between the degree of Jewish orthodoxy and the frequency of heart attack among 10,000 municipal employees followed over five years in Israel.[57] He found that Jews who were more orthodox in their religious belief and practice experienced lower rates of heart attack.

Some time later, it was discovered that members of certain religious groups had lower mortality from heart disease than persons in the general population. In 1978, Phillips and colleagues[58] found lower death rates from coronary heart disease among Seventh-Day Adventists; not long after that, Lyon and colleagues[59] reported similar findings in Mormons. While these investigators explained their findings as due to better diet, less smoking, and other health behaviors, they could not exclude the possibility that greater religiousness (which caused subjects to comply with these behavioral restrictions) played a role.

More recently, Friedlander and colleagues[60] reported that the risk of heart attack for men who were not religious was four to seven times higher than that of religious men, even after taking into account the usual risk factors for heart disease. In 1993, Goldbourt and colleagues[61] published, in the widely respected journal *Cardiology*, a 23-year follow-up on over 10,000 civil employees involved in Medalie's cardiovascular study mentioned earlier. Again, these investigators found that greater Jewish orthodoxy was associated with a lower death rate from coronary heart disease (see Figure 6.5), a difference that persisted after taking into account age, blood pressure, cholesterol, smoking, diabetes, weight, and baseline heart disease. Thus, evidence is mounting for a link between lower rates of heart disease and both church attendance and greater religiousness.

One of the most significant mortality studies to date was published in the January 1995 issue of *Psychosomatic Medicine*. Thomas Oxman and colleagues[62] at Dartmouth followed 232 patients for six months after open-heart surgery, examining psychological, social, and health factors that predicted mortality. Persons who did not derive strength and comfort from religion were over three times as likely (odds ratio 3.25) to die as those who did receive comfort from religion. Likewise, those who did

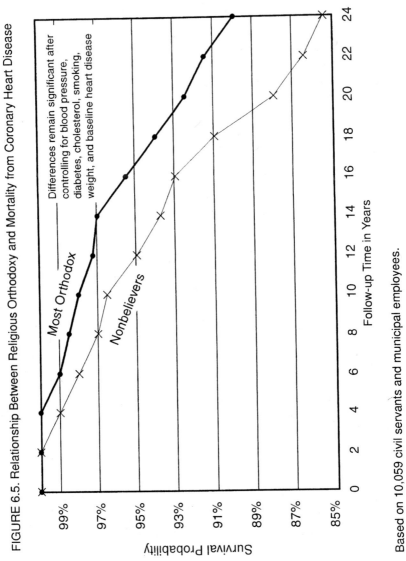

FIGURE 6.5. Relationship Between Religious Orthodoxy and Mortality from Coronary Heart Disease

Differences remain significant after controlling for blood pressure, diabetes, cholesterol, smoking, weight, and baseline heart disease

Most Orthodox

Nonbelievers

Survival Probability

Follow-up Time in Years

Based on 10,059 civil servants and municipal employees.

Source: Kaplan-Meier life table curves; adapted from Goldbourt et al. (1993). *Cardiology* 82:100-121.

not participate in social groups were over four times as likely to die (odds ratio 4.26) as those who did. Even after controlling for a multitude of health factors (previous cardiac surgery, physical functioning, age, and so forth), patients who neither participated in social groups nor derived comfort from religion were 12 times more likely to die than those who were religiously and socially active (see Figure 6.6).

Finally, in a controversial and yet-to-be replicated study, Randolph Byrd examined the therapeutic effects of intercessory prayer in patients hospitalized on the coronary care unit of a large metropolitan hospital.[63] Byrd, then a cardiologist at San Francisco General Hospital, randomly assigned 393 patients to

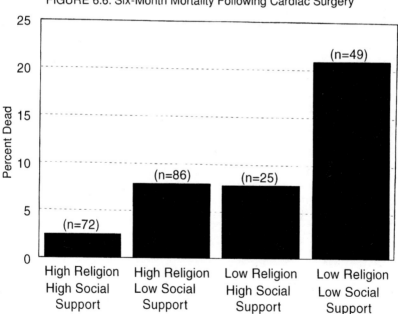

FIGURE 6.6. Six-Month Mortality Following Cardiac Surgery

Based on 232 patients at Dartmouth Medical Center in Lebanon, New Hampshire.

Source: Adapted from Oxman et al. (1995). *Psychosomatic Medicine* 57:5-15. Reprinted by permission.

one of two groups. One group of 192 patients received intercessory prayer by Christian prayer groups located outside the hospital. The other group of 201 patients (the control group) were not
prayed for by the prayer groups. The prayer groups did not know
the patients they were praying for. Neither the patients nor their
physicians knew that they were being prayed for. In a finding that
shocked the scientific world, the prayed-for patients experienced
significantly better medical outcomes than did patients without
prayer, including less ventilator assistance, and fewer antibiotics
and other medications. Several investigators around the country
are now trying to replicate this study. None of the direct or
indirect mechanisms described above can be invoked to explain
this result, which if true, was either the result of some type of
supernatural intervention or was based on something like the "new
physics" that has been so popular in New Age circles recently.

## *CANCER*

Cancer is the leading cause of death in adults age 25 to 64,
with nearly 150 out of every 100,000 Americans in this age range
dying from cancer each year (30 percent of which are linked to
smoking and 35 percent to diet).[64,65] A wide range of studies
have found lower rates of cancer among members of certain
religious groups (see Figure 6.7). To date, at least 16 studies have
examined cancer rates in Mormons,[66-71] Seventh-Day Adventists,[72-75] Jews,[76-79] Hutterites,[80] and Amish.[81] Except for the
Jewish studies, all found lower cancer rates in members of these
religious groups compared with persons in the general population. In the Jewish studies, findings were mixed. Jewish women
tended to have higher rates of cancer than did women from other
religious groups, whereas Jewish men tended to have lower rates
of cancer (primarily lung cancer) than non-Jewish men. Jewish
women, on the other hand, experienced lower rates of cervical
and breast cancer than non-Jewish women. Lower rates of cervi-

FIGURE 6.7. Death Rates from Cancer, by Religious Group

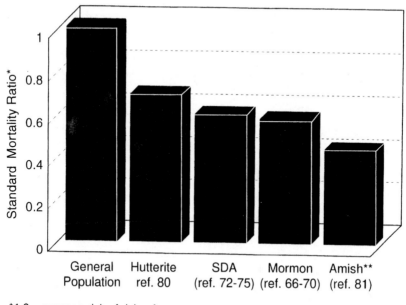

*1.0 = average risk of dying from cancer.
**Males age 40-69 only.

cal cancer in Jewish women have long been attributed to the Jewish male practice of circumcision.

More recently, Dwyer and colleagues[71] examined the effects of concentration density of different religious groups on county cancer mortality rates, speculating that the dietary and behavioral restrictions placed on religious adherents might benefit not only them, but also persons in the surrounding community who were not of the same faith. They found that counties with the highest concentrations of conservative Protestants, moderate Protestants, or Mormons had the lowest cancer mortality rates, whereas communities with greater concentrations of liberal Protestants, Catholics, or Jews, had higher cancer mortality rates. These findings were independent of demographic, environmental, and regional factors known to affect cancer mortality.

The investigators concluded that religion does have an impact at the community level. In other words, communities with high concentrations of persons from more conservative religious traditions may derive health benefits from a reduced exposure to and social disapproval of habits and behaviors known to increase the risk of cancer. Again, it is difficult to sort out whether the reduced cancer risk is due primarily to healthy lifestyles, diet, and avoidance of alcohol and smoking, or if it is due to an underlying factor such as "religious commitment" that causes people to conform to such behavioral restrictions.

## ALL-CAUSE MORTALITY

Does religious commitment prolong life? The above studies suggest that it might by protecting persons from cardiovascular diseases and cancer. A number of studies have examined the association between religiousness and overall mortality (death from any cause).[2] Twenty-three studies have examined the association between religiousness and mortality (excluding studies that examine denomination only). Of those, the vast majority have found a positive association between greater religiousness and lower death rates. The longer persons were followed in such studies, the more likely that researchers identified a positive effect.[2] Four studies examined death from suicide; all found lower suicide among the more religious.[16-19] Four studies examined survival among clergy; again, all four studies found that clergy live longer than persons in the general population.[82-85] Eight studies examined the effect of church attendance on survival. Five of the eight found that those who attend church more frequently live longer.[55,86-89] While it may be true that those who are healthy are more *able* to attend church, this is not the whole story. Several of these studies have taken disability level into account and still found that the more religiously involved live longer.

Religiousness may increase survival even for those who are already severely ill. This is what Zuckerman and colleagues[87] found in their study of predictors of mortality for a population of 400 elderly residents of New Haven, Connecticut. Religiousness at the start of the study was measured by frequency of church attendance, degree of self-professed religiousness, and the utilization of religion as a source of comfort and strength. The investigators followed subjects for a two-year period and at the end of this time examined the characteristics of persons who had died. They found that subjects who were more religious survived longer, even after taking into account both health and sex. The effect was especially noticeable among those who were sick at the start of the study. Among the sick who were religious, only 19 percent of men and 11 percent of women died; among the sick who were not religious, 42 percent of men and 20 percent of women died.

These Yale researchers concluded that religiousness had a protective effect against mortality among the elderly in poor health. The element of religiousness that had the greatest effect on mortality was not church attendance, but *comfort derived from religion*. In several studies above, then, we have found that persons who depend on and receive comfort from their religious beliefs experience both better mental health and longer survival.

## SUMMARY

The research to date, then, appears to show that persons who are more religious are physically healthier and tend to live longer than those who are not religious. This does not necessarily mean that religion causes people to be healthier, but it provides substantive evidence that this may be the case. Indeed, we have described a model based on natural mechanisms by which these effects on health could be conveyed (see Figure 6.2). Well known are the physical health effects of strong social support, better mental health, healthier lifestyles, avoidance of alcohol and smoking, early recognition of disease and greater compliance with treatment, and these have been increasingly linked to religious beliefs and practices. More research is clearly needed to (1) determine if greater religiousness truly causes better physical health, (2) discover what particular aspects of religion provide such protective effects, and (3) identify what aspects of health are most sensitive to the effects of religious involvement.

## REFERENCE NOTES

1. Levin, J.S., and P.L. Schiller. (1987). Is there a religious factor in health? *Journal of Religion and Health* 26:9-36.

2. McCullough, M.E., Larson, D.B., Koenig, H.G., Milano, M.G. Systematic review of published research assessing the relationship between religious commitment and mortality, 1987-1995. *Journal of the American Medical Association,* in submission.

3. Koenig, H.G. (1996). A prevention model explaining religion's effects on health. Presented at symposium "Religion, Social and Environmental Influences on Health" at the *American Association for the Advancement of Science* annual meeting, Baltimore, Maryland, February 11, 1996.

4. Naguib, S.M., P.B. Beiser, and G.W. Comstock. (1968). Response to a program of screening for cervical cancer. *Public Health Reports* 83(12):990-998.

5. Van Reek, J., and M.J. Drop. (1986). Cigarette smoking in the U.S.A.: Sociocultural influences. *Rev Epidemiol Sante Publique* 34(3):168-173.

6. Cobb, S. (1976). Social support as a moderator of life stress. *Journal of Psychosomatic Medicine* 38:300-314.

7. Cassel, J. (1976). The contribution of the social environment to host resistance. *American Journal of Epidemiology* 104:107-123.

8. Antonovsky, A. (1979). *Health, Stress, and Coping.* San Francisco: Jossey-Bass.

9. Durkheim, E. (1951). *Suicide.* New York: The Free Press.

10. Berkman, L.F., and S.L. Syme. (1979). Social networks, host resistance, and mortality: A nine-year follow-up study of Alameda County residents. *American Journal of Epidemiology* 109:2,186-204.

11. Blazer, D. (1982). Social support and mortality in an elderly community population. *American Journal of Epidemiology* 115:684-694.

12. Broadhead, W.E., B.H. Kaplan, S.A. James, E.H. Wagner, V.J. Schoenbach, R. Grimson, S. Heyden, G. Tibblin, and S.H. Gehlbach. (1983). The epidemiologic evidence for a relationship between social support and health. *American Journal of Epidemiology* 117:521-537.

13. Cohen, J.B., and J.A. Brody. (1981). The epidemiological importance of psychosocial factors in longevity. *American Journal of Epidemiology* 114:451-461.

14. House, J.S., K.R. Landis, and D. Umberson. (1988). Social relationships and health. *Science* 241:540.

15. Spiegel, D., J.R. Bloom, H.C. Kraemer, and E. Gottheil. (1989). Effect of psychosocial treatment on survival of patients with metastatic breast cancer. *Lancet* (no. 8668):888-891.

16. Martin, W.T. (1984). Religiosity and United States suicide rates, 1972-1978. *Journal of Clinical Psychology* 40(5):1166-1169.

17. Stack, S. (1983). The effect of religious commitment on suicide: A cross-national analysis. *Journal of Health and Social Behavior* (pp. 362-374).

18. Stack, S. (1983). The effect of religiosity on suicide. *Journal for the Scientific Study of Religion* 22:239-252.

19. Breault, K.D., and K. Barkey. (1982). A comparative analysis of Durkheim's theory of egoistic suicide. *The Sociological Quarterly* 23:321-331.

20. Restak, R.M. (1989). The brain, depression, and the immune system. *Journal of Clinical Psychiatry* 50 (5, Suppl.):23-25.

21. Breier, A., M. Albus, D. Pickar, T.P. Zahn, O.M. Wolkowitz, and S.M. Paul. (1987). Controllable and uncontrollable stress in humans: Alterations in mood and neuroendocrine and psychophysiological function. *American Journal of Psychiatry* 144:1419-1425.

22. Ader, R. (1981). *Psychoneuroimmunology.* NY: Academic Press.

23. Schleifer, S.J., S.E. Keller, M. Camerino, J.C. Thornton, and M. Stein. (1983). Suppression of lymphocyte stimulation following bereavement. *Journal of the American Medical Association* 250:274-377.

24. Bartrop, R.W., L. Lazarus, E. Luckhurst, L.G. Kiloh, and R. Penny. (1977). Depressed lymphocyte function after bereavement. *Lancet* (April 16, 1977), pp. 834-836.

25. Irwin, M., T. Patterson, T.L. Smith, C. Caldwell, S.A. Brown, C. Gillin, and I. Grant. (1990). Reduction of immune function in life stress and depression. *Biological Psychiatry* 27:22-30.

26. Shekelle, R.B., W.J. Raynor, A.M. Ostfeld, D.C. Garron, L.A. Bicliauskas, S.C. Lu, C. Maliza, O. Paul. (1981). Psychological depression and 17-year risk of death from cancer. *Psychosomatic Medicine* 43:117-125.

27. Greer, S. (1983). Cancer and the mind. *British Journal of Psychiatry* 143:535-543.

28. Hambling, J. (1951). Emotions and symptoms in essential hypertension. *British Journal of Medical Psychology* 24:242-250.

29. Adler, R., K. MacRitchie, and G.L. Engel. (1971). Psychologic processes and ischemic stroke (occlusive cerebrovascular disease): Observations on 32 men with 35 strokes. *Psychosomatic Medicine* 33:1-29.

30. Rosengren, A., G. Tibblin, and L. Wilhelmsen. (1991). Self-perceived psychological stress and incidence of coronary artery disease in middle-aged men. *American Journal of Cardiology* 68:1171-1175.

31. Cobb, S., and R.M. Rose. (1973). Hypertension, peptic ulcer, and diabetes in air traffic controllers. *Journal of the American Medical Association* 224:489-492.

32. Engel, G.L. (1955). Studies of ulcerative colitis: III. The nature of psychologic processes. *American Journal of Medicine* (August 1955):231-256.

33. Rovner, B.W., P. German, and L.J. Brant, et al. (1991). Depression and mortality in nursing homes. *Journal of the American Medical Association* 265:993-996.

34. Frasure-Smith, N., F. Lesperance, and M. Talajic. (1993). Depression following myocardial infarction. *Journal of the American Medical Association* 270:1819-1825.

35. Burt, V.L., Whelton, P., Roccella, E.J. (1995). Prevalence of hypertension in the U.S. adult population: Results from the Third National Health and Nutrition Examination Survey, 1988-1991. *Hypertension* 25:305-313.

36. Weiner, H. (1979). *The Psychobiology of Hypertension.* New York: Elsevier.

37. Jacob, R.G., H.C. Kramer, and W.S. Agras. (1977). Relaxation therapy in the treatment of hypertension. *Archives of General Psychiatry* 34:1417-1427.

38. Brody, D.S. (1980). Psychological distress and hypertension control. *Journal of Human Stress* March 1980: 2-6.

39. Taylor, C.B., and S.P. Fortman. (1983). Psychosomatic illness review: Hypertension. *Psychosomatics* 24:433-448.

40. Linden, W., and M. Feuerstein. (1981). Essential hypertension and social coping behavior. *Journal of Human Stress* March 1981: 28-34.

41. Larson, D.B., H.G. Koenig, B.H. Kaplan, R.S. Greenberg, E. Logue, and H.A. Tyroler. (1989). The impact of religion on men's blood pressure. *Journal of Religion and Health* 28:265-278.

42. Koenig, H.G., D.O. Moberg, and J.N. Kvale. (1988). Religious activities and attitudes of older adults in a geriatric assessment clinic. *Journal of the American Geriatrics Society* 36:362-374.

43. Livingston, I.L., D.M. Levine, and R.D. Moore. (1991). Social integration and black intraracial variation in blood pressure. *Ethnicity and Disease* 1:135-149.

44. Graham, T.W., B.H. Kaplan, J.C. Cornoni-Huntley, S.A. James, C. Becker, C.G. Hames, and S. Heyden. (1978). Frequency of church attendance and blood pressure elevation. *Journal of Behavioral Medicine* 1(1):37-43.

45. Hutchinson, J. (1986). Association between stress and blood pressure variation in a Caribbean population. *American Journal of Physical Anthropology* 71:69-79.

46. Walsh, A. (1980). The prophylactic effect of religion on blood pressure levels among a sample of immigrants. *Social Sciences and Medicine* 14B:59-63.

47. Levin, J.S., and K.S. Markides. (1985). Religion and health in Mexican Americans. *Journal of Religion and Health* 24:60-69.

48. Scotch, N.A. (1963). Sociocultural factors in the epidemiology of Zulu hypertension. *American Journal of Public Health* 53:1205-1213.

49. Armstrong, B., A. Merwyk, and H. Coates. (1977). Blood pressure in Seventh-Day Adventist vegetarians. *American Journal of Epidemiology* 105:444-449.

50. National Center for Health Statistics. (1990). *Health, United States, 1989 and Prevention Profile*. DHHS Pub. No. (PHS) 90-1232. Hyattsville, MD: U.S. Department of Health and Human Services.

51. Feigenson, J. (1979). Stroke rehabilitation: Effectiveness, benefits, and cost. *Stroke* 10:1-4.

52. Colantonio, A., S.V. Kasl, and A.M. Ostfeld. (1992). Depressive symptoms and other psychosocial factors as predictors of stroke in the elderly. *American Journal of Epidemiology* 136:884-894.

53. *Healthy People 2000*. (1991). National Health Promotion and Disease Prevention: U.S. Department of Health and Human Services, Public Health Service, DHHS Publication No. (PHS) 91-50212, (p. 394).

54. Wardwell, W.I., C.B. Bahnson, and H.S. Caron. (1963). Social and psychological factors in coronary heart disease. *Journal of Health and Human Behavior* 4:154-165.

55. Comstock, G.W. (1971). Fatal arteriosclerotic heart disease, water hardness at home, and socioeconomic characteristics. *American Journal of Epidemiology* 94:1-10.

56. Comstock, G.W., and K.B. Partridge. (1972). Church attendance and health. *Journal of Chronic Disease* 25:665-672.

57. Medalie, J.H., H.A. Kahn, H.N. Neufeld, E. Riss, and U. Goldbourt. (1973). Five-year myocardial infarction incidence: II. Association of single variables to age and birthplace. *Journal of Chronic Disease* 26:329-349.

58. Phillips, R.L., F.R. Lemon, W.L. Beeson, and J.W. Kuzma. (1978). Coronary heart disease mortality among Seventh-Day Adventists with differing dietary habits: A preliminary report. *The American Journal of Clinical Nutrition* 31: S191-S198.

59. Lyon, J.L., H.P. Wetzler, J.W. Gardner, M.R. Klauber, and R.R. Williams. (1978). Cardiovascular mortality in Mormons and non-Mormons in Utah, 1969-1971. *American Journal of Epidemiology* 108:5,357-366.

60. Friedlander, Y., J.D. Kark, and Y. Stein. (1986). Religious orthodoxy and myocardial infarction in Jerusalem: A case control study. *International Journal of Cardiology* 10:33-41.

61. Goldbourt, U., S. Yaari, and J.H. Medalie. (1993). Factors predictive of long-term coronary heart disease mortality among 10,059 male Israeli civil servants and municipal employees: A 23-year mortality follow-up in the Israeli Ischemic Heart Disease study. *Cardiology* 82:100-121.

62. Oxman, T.E., D.H. Freeman, and E.D. Manheimer. (1995). Lack of social participation or religious strength and comfort as risk factors for death after cardiac surgery in the elderly. *Psychosomatic Medicine* 57:5-15.

63. Byrd, R.C. (1988). Positive therapeutic effects of intercessory prayer in a coronary care unit population. *Southern Medical Journal* 81:826-829.

64. *Healthy People 2000*. (1991). National Health Promotion and Disease Prevention: U.S. Department of Health and Human Services, Public Health Services, DHHS Publication No. (PHS) 91-50212, (p. 19).

65. Ibid., p. 416

66. Enstrom, J.E. (1975). Cancer mortality among Mormons. *Cancer* 36:825-841.

67. Lyon, J.L., M.R. Klauber, J.W. Gardner, and C.R. Smart. (1976). Cancer incidence in Mormons and non-Mormons in Utah, 1966-1970. *New England Journal of Medicine* 294:129-133.

68. Jarvis, G.K. (1977). Mormon mortality rates in Canada. *Social Biology* 24: 294-302.

69. Lyon, J.L., J.W. Gardner, M.R. Klauber, and C.R. Smart. (1977). Low cancer incidence and mortality in Utah. *Cancer* 39:2608-2618.

70. Enstrom, J.E. (1978). Cancer and total mortality among active Mormons. *Cancer* 42:1943-1951.

71. Dwyer, J.W., L.L. Clarke, and M.K. Miller. (1990). The effect of religious concentration and affiliation on county cancer mortality rates. *Journal of Health and Social Behavior* 31:185-202.

72. Phillips, R.L., J.W. Kuzma, W.L. Beeson, and T. Lotz. (1980). Influence of selection versus lifestyle on risk of fatal cancer and cardiovascular disease among Seventh-Day Adventists. *American Journal of Epidemiology* 112:296-314.

73. Phillips, R.L., and D.A. Snowden. (1983). Association of meat and coffee use with cancers of the large bowel, breast, and prostate among Seventh-Day Adventists: Preliminary results. *Cancer Research* 43 (Supplement):2403s-2408s.

74. Berkel, J., and F. deWaard. (1983). Mortality pattern and life expectancy of Seventh-Day Adventists in the Netherlands. *International Journal of Epidemiology* 12:455-459.

75. Zollinger, T.W., R.L. Phillips, and J.W. Kuzma. (1984). Breast cancer survival rates among Seventh-Day Adventists and non-Seventh-Day Adventists. *American Journal of Epidemiology* 119:503-509.

76. Seidman, H. (1970). Cancer death rates by site and sex for religious and socioeconomic groups in New York City. *Environmental Research* 3:234-250.

77. MacMahon, B. (1960). The ethnic distribution of cancer mortality in New York City, 1955. *Acta-Unio Internationale Contra Cancrum* 16:1716-1724.

78. Herman, B., and P.E. Enterline. (1970). Lung cancer among the Jews and non-Jews of Pittsburgh, Pennsylvania, 1953-1967: Mortality rates and cigarette-smoking behavior. *American Journal of Epidemiology* 91:355-367.

79. Greenwald, P., R.F. Korns, P.C. Nasca, and P.E. Wolfgang. (1975). Cancer in United States Jews. *Cancer Research* 35:3507-3512.

80. Martin, A.O., J.K. Dunn, J.L. Simpson, C.L. Olsen, S. Kemel, M. Grace, S. Elias, G.E. Sarto, B. Smalley, and A.G. Steinberg. (1980). Cancer mortality in a human isolate. *Journal of the National Cancer Institute* 65:1109-1113.

81. Hamman, R.F., J.I. Barancik, and A.M. Lilienfeld. (1981). Patterns of mortality in the old order Amish: I. Background and major causes of death. *American Journal of Epidemiology* 114:845-861.

82. Ogata, M., M. Ikeda, and M. Kuratsune. (1984). Mortality among Japanese Zen priests. *Journal of Epidemiology and Community Health* 38:161-166.

83. Locke, F.B., and H. King. (1980). Mortality among Baptist clergymen. *Journal of Chronic Diseases* 33:581-590.

84. Madigan, F.C. (1961). Role satisfactions and length of life in a closed population. *American Journal of Sociology* 67:640-649.

85. King, H., and F.B. Locke. (1980). American White Protestant clergy as a low-risk population for mortality research. *Journal of the National Cancer Institute* 65:1115-1124.

86. Schoenback, V.J., B.H. Kaplan, L. Fredman, and D.G. Kleinbaum. (1986). Social ties and morality in Evans County, Georgia. *American Journal of Epidemiology* 123:577-591.

87. Zuckerman, D.M., S.V. Kasl, and A.M. Ostfeld. (1984). Psychosocial predictors of mortality among the elderly poor. The role of religion, well-being, and social contacts. *American Journal of Epidemiology* 119:410-423.

88. Comstock, G.W., and J.A. Tonascia. (1977). Education and morality in Washington County, Maryland. *Journal of Health and Social Behavior* 18:54-61.

89. House, J.S., C. Robbins, and H.L. Metzner. (1982). The association of social relationships and activities with mortality: Prospective evidence from the Tecumseh Community Health Study. *American Journal of Epidemiology* 116:123-140.

# Chapter 7

# Conclusions and Reanalysis

Based on the research described previously, we can come to some tentative and cautious conclusions about the relationship between religion and health. One conclusion we can make with a high degree of confidence is that religion, particularly that based in traditional Judeo-Christian belief and practice, does not have a negative influence on health. This, of course, excludes religious cults similar to those involved in the Jonestown massacre and Waco disaster, as well as other deviant religious groups operating on the fringe of society or outside of an established religious tradition on the fringe of society. There is simply no solid research that supports a negative influence on mental or physical health for church attendance, prayer, scripture reading, or devout religious commitment, particularly when these occur in the context of an established Judeo-Christian religious tradition. What about the positive effects of religious belief and practice on mental and physical health?

## *EFFECTS ON MENTAL HEALTH*

In general, devout religiousness and frequent involvement in both private and public religious activities are associated with better mental health. More specifically:

- A large segment of the American population (as high as 20 to 40 percent) says that religion is one of the most important factors that enable them to cope with stressful life circumstances.[1-7]

• The use of religion as a coping behavior is associated with higher self-esteem[8] and less depression,[2,9] particularly among persons who are physically disabled. It can also predict who will and will not become depressed over time.[2]

• Devout religious commitment (intrinsic religiosity, in particular) is associated with lower rates of depression,[10-12] quicker recovery from depression,[3] greater well-being and morale,[13] higher self-esteem,[10] an internal locus of control,[14] marital adjustment and satisfaction,[15-20] and more rapid adaptation in caregivers of patients with dementia or end-stage cancer.[21]

• Frequent church or synagogue attendance is associated with a 40 to 50 percent reduction in the risk of depression,[22,23] lower rates of suicide,[24,25] lower rates of anxiety disorder,[26] lower rates of alcoholism and drug use,[27-31] higher social support,[32] greater well-being,[13,33] happiness,[34] adjustment,[34] usefulness,[34] higher self-esteem,[35] higher life satisfaction,[36-40] and predicts positive affect and mood 12 years later among younger adults.[41]

• Private religious activities, such as prayer and scripture reading, are associated with greater well-being,[13,37] greater life satisfaction,[27,42] less death anxiety,[43] and lower rates of alcoholism and drug use.[27]

• Interventions for depression and anxiety disorder that integrate religion with psychotherapy induce recovery quicker than secular techniques alone.[44,45]

## EFFECTS ON PHYSICAL HEALTH

The effects of religious beliefs and activities on physical health are similar to those on mental health. In general, persons who are religiously involved are healthier than those who are not. More specifically:

- At any given level of chronic illness, men who are more religious perceive their ability to function as higher than those who are not religious.[46]
- Frequent church attendance predicts lower levels of physical disability among older persons at one, two, and three years of followup.[47]
- Religiousness predicts more rapid recovery from hip fracture (in terms of meters walked and ambulation status at hospital discharge).[9]
- Intensity of religious belief and church attendance is associated with lower pain levels perceived by patients with end-stage cancer.[48]
- Religiousness is associated with lower rates of cigarette smoking.[49]
- Frequent church attendance and importance of religion are associated with lower blood pressure, both systolic and diastolic.[50-56]
- Frequent church attendance (weekly or more often) is associated with a lower risk of stroke in controlled analyses.[57]
- Religious orthodoxy and frequent church attendance are associated with fewer myocardial infarctions and a lower death rate from coronary artery disease.[58-65]
- Religious coping is associated with both a lower death rate following cardiac surgery[66] and lower mortality in general.[67]
- Intercessory prayer has been shown to result in lower cardiovascular complications following admission to a coronary care unit, although the mechanism of this effect (if true) remains unknown.[68]
- Certain religious groups have lower rates of cancer due to diet, lifestyle, and probably level of religious commit-

ment[69-84]; this protective effect appears to generalize to entire communities, affecting even those not of the same faith.[74]

- Persons who are more religiously involved appear to have lower overall mortality in more than 80% of studies that have examined this association.[85]

## PATHOLOGICAL ASPECTS OF RELIGION REANALYZED

The adverse effects of religious belief and behavior on health appear to have been overemphasized by health professionals like Freud, Ellis, and Watters. In general, we have seen that traditional beliefs and practices based in the Judeo-Christian religious tradition do not have a negative influence on mental or physical health. The results of much systematic research, in fact, demonstrate that people who are more religiously involved demonstrate better mental and physical health. This does not mean, however, that religious belief and practice *cannot be used in a destructive way*. While the neurotic and pathological uses of religion are not widespread nor characteristic of the vast majority of Americans who are religious, they do occur in individual cases and so deserve mention here to round out and balance our discussion. Paul Pruyser has examined the negative uses of religion[86]; among these are the following:

- Sacrifice of the intellect
- Rationalization for hatred, aggression, and prejudice
- Thought control and promotion of excessive dependency
- Surrender of agency, dissociation, and disavowal
- Justification for being judgmental and insensitive to situations
- Displacement to the body (self-punishment, asceticism)
- Obsessional thinking (sin and guilt)
- Reinforcement of undesirable character traits

I will now briefly discuss each of these neurotic uses of religion. Religious doctrines by themselves are seldom pathological; rather, it is the neurotic tendencies of those who *use religion* that make it pathological for them.

### Sacrifice of the Intellect

Neurotic beliefs often separate and oppose both faith and reason. Such beliefs demand the ultimate sacrifice of reason and encourage a total dependence on "blind faith." This often occurs when specific biblical verses are pulled out of context, overemphasized, and not balanced with the rest of scripture. Certain Judeo-Christian teachings do require "believing without seeing," for *reason* itself cannot be an idol that comes before God. Nevertheless, scriptures also teach that persons are accountable for the things they do and believe, and that "prophesies" from others should always be "tested." Thus, widely accepted Judeo-Christian teachings seldom promote a total sacrifice of the intellect, but rather a balance of reason and faith. Some individuals with poor ego functioning, whose beliefs are easily swayed by others, however, may be duped into suspending all reason and intelligence and following blindly after "such singularly undeserving persons as an obese adolescent from India or a right-wing agitator from South Korea, both of whom go blatantly to the pockets of their followers" (p. 332).[86] Here again, the problem is often the individual's neurotic or manipulative use of religion, rather than the teachings themselves. In such persons, faith frequently becomes confused with fantasy and wishful thinking.

### Rationalization for Hatred, Aggression, and Prejudice

Many deeply wounded individuals carry bitterness and a desire for revenge within them. Their insecurity and low self-esteem prevents them from assertively confronting those who have hurt them. Instead, their anger is repressed and diverted into more acceptable channels of release, one of which may be religion. As religious people, however, they seldom demonstrate the love, acceptance, and mercy that is central to their faith. Rather, they focus on denouncing others who believe differently than they do and accuse those outside of their small group of being lost sinners, belonging to the devil, and deserving eternal punishment in hell. Such persons use religion as a way to release their hatred and aggressive impulses onto others, cleverly cloaking them in theological terms that are expressed with pious, better-than-thou attitudes.

### Thought Control and Promotion of Excessive Dependency

Religion can be used as a tool to control the thoughts and behaviors of others, particularly those who are excessively dependent and needy of approval by others. By paying special attention to these needy and vulnerable individuals, a charismatic religious figure can easily recruit them into his or her group and convince them that he or she is speaking for God and therefore demands total obedience. Any type of free thinking or debate is discouraged. The religious leader begins thinking for his or her followers. Followers are often separated and isolated from contact with persons outside their small group. Outsiders are seen by the group as infidels who are persecuting them. This further reinforces ties within the group and separates members from outside influences. Religious leaders, operating outside of any established religious tradition with a hierarchy of leadership, are typically accountable to no one higher than their own self. Narcissistic and power-thirsty, as such persons tend to be, they take on a "messiah complex" and see themselves as "God's chosen one." Their followers also begin seeing them in this way and obey without questioning. In a sense, the leader takes the place of

God. Jim Jones and David Koresh are examples of religious figures who acquired almost total mind control over their followers.

## Surrender of Agency, Dissociation, and Disavowal

Religion can be used to justify a loss of control over the self. Persons with weak ego strength and poorly formed sense of self may excuse their negative or destructive actions as being due to the influence of an evil or malevolent force outside of themselves (e.g., "the devil made me do it"). Here, the person surrenders ego control and is "temporarily swept away by a regression in which the self is no longer held accountable" (p. 336).[86] This "surrender of agency" can result in a completely dissociated state in which time is lost and activities cannot be recalled. The main point is that persons lose accountability for their actions–a process nowhere condoned in traditional Judeo-Christian teachings.

## Justification for Being Judgmental

Religion can be used by insecure and emotionally unstable persons to make them feel significant and part of a group that is "chosen" or has special knowledge that others outside their own group do not have. These individuals carefully scrutinize the actions of others and piously judge their behaviors against the most rigorous standards–standards which they themselves cannot usually keep. By judging others as base and unworthy, these persons feel better about themselves. Judgments of others are usually made through the often unconscious biases of the judger's own past, are typically based on a superficial understanding of the judged person's circumstances, and often show a singular lack of sensitivity to and respect for the other as a unique individual. As noted before, such judgments are often justified by the misuse and overemphasis of certain religious scriptures, while ignoring other scriptures meant to balance them, such as "Judge not, that ye be not judged."

## Displacement to the Body

Here, religion is used in order to act out deeply rooted masochistic tendencies. Conflict-laden urges are thus displaced onto the body. According to Pruyser,[85]

> It is one thing to accept torture as it comes, for the sake of principle; it is another thing to seek martyrdom as an end in itself and trap oneself into it. Undemanded and self-imposed, such suffering bespeaks a wish for self-destruction either by masochistic urges or as a necessary atonement for some real or imagined wrongdoing which an implacable conscience demands. (p. 341)[85]

Strict asceticism may be practiced in the name of holiness. Guilt-ridden, self-hating persons neglect or abuse their bodies and justify these actions by pointing to religious doctrines stressing that bodily existence is of no significance or that parts of the body are evil and deserving of whipping, starving, or some other form of severe discipline. Again, these persons completely neglect other central teachings that emphasize a need to respect and care for the body as a "temple of the Holy Spirit."

## Obsessional Thinking

Certain psychiatric disorders are characterized by obsessional preoccupation with a thought or idea that evokes anxiety or guilt. Such obsessions are often accompanied by compulsive, repetitive activities meant to relieve the anxiety aroused by the thought. Religious beliefs and activities nicely fit into the psychopathology of such persons. Preoccupation over real or imagined sins is followed by repeated acts of penance to compensate for the misdeed. Incessant prayers, compulsive church-going, or repetitive visits to the confessional may be seen by a religious congregation as acts of genuine devotion. However, the individual is driven by deep anxieties and insecurities, rather than a love for God or for holiness. Such people can be detected by the increase in anxiety they experience when they cannot perform these religious duties. Neither love of God nor love of man comes before their rituals. Again, it is their mental illness that drives these behaviors, not the religious doctrines they espouse.

### Reinforcement of Undesirable Character Traits

Personality traits are frequently egosyntonic—in other words, persons accept these traits as part of themselves, often prizing them as necessary and desirable. This holds true for both positive *and negative* character traits. Religious doctrines can be used to justify or reinforce certain negative character traits. For example, the narcissist may need to view himself or herself as "special" and deserving of others' attention and praise. Religious scriptures may be used to "prove" that he or she is called and anointed by God to carry out some great mission. If disconnected from reality, these notions may develop into frank delusions. Likewise, self-righteous persons may find proofs in scripture that their views are the only correct ones and that everyone else is wrong, thus feeding their own self-esteem by their judgment and condemnation. Other examples of religion being used to reinforce negative character traits include the dishonest or fraudulent individuals who use religion to manipulate others for financial gain, or the suspicious, hypervigilant person who uses religion as a shield to keep others at a distance by hurling scriptures at them.

For a more detailed discussion on the pathological uses of religion, see *Religious Factors in Mental Illness* by Wayne Oates (NY: Association Press, 1955) and *Churches That Abuse* by Ronald Enroth (Grand Rapids, MI: Zondervan, 1992).

### Conclusion and Synthesis

In most of these neurotic uses of religion, as I have said before, it is the person's insecurity or mental disturbance—not the religious doctrine–that drives behavior. Religion is often used to justify pathological tendencies. When this happens, persons pull selected religious scriptures or Bible verses out of context and overemphasize them, while ignoring more central religious doctrines meant to counterbalance these teachings and prevent excesses. Thus, it is the misuse and abuse of religion that most neurotic manifestations of it reflect. These neurotic uses of religion are common in small religious groups or cults that exist outside of the established, mainstream Judeo-Christian traditions, in which the hierarchy of leadership is often limited to a single, all-powerful leader who is responsible to no one but the god whom he or she has created in the image of his or her own self. The controls and balances that normally operate when groups have input from those outside the group are absent, allowing extremes and excesses to proceed unchecked.

While there is a grain of truth in what Freud and other mental health specialists have been saying about religion, it is a misunderstood truth. Because mental health professionals primarily see patients with psychopathologies, they are more likely than anyone else to see the neurotic uses of religion. We cannot conclude, however, from this limited clinical exposure, that religion is the cause of the patients' neuroses or that such pathological uses of religion are characteristic of its use by the vast majority of those in established religious traditions. Indeed, the research shows quite the opposite. Most persons employ religion in a healthy way to cope with real-life stresses and existential issues, and do so quite successfully. Persons who use religion in a mature way may infrequently need the expertise of psychologists and psychiatrists. Consequently, these professionals seldom see religion used in this way. Even when religion is used effectively and adaptively, mental health specialists may not recognize it as such, due either to a lack of training in this area or, sometimes, to a lack of healthy religion in their own lives.

We have attempted elsewhere[87] to distill some of the healthy components of the Christian belief system and describe how the practice of these principles can meet many basic psychological and spiritual needs. It is usually the immature forms of religious expression that lend themselves to neurotic use. Mature employments of religion that emphasize love, forgiveness, acceptance, mercy and compassion are difficult to neuroticize. Discussing how we might distinguish neurotic from healthy use of religion, Nancy Andreasen (now editor-in-chief of the *American Journal of Psychiatry*) as a psychiatry resident at the University of Iowa in the early 1970s wrote,[88]

> Although there are fancier and more refined criteria, ultimately the capacity to function productively and well is perhaps the best; here Freud's use of *lieben und arbeiten*, the biblical dictum "by their fruits ye shall know them," and common sense are all in agreement. (p. 157)

## *SUMMARY*

Cross-sectional, longitudinal, and intervention studies have demonstrated positive effects for religious belief and practice on both mental and physical health. This research does not support opinions based on clinical experience forwarded by Freud, Ellis, Watters, and other health professionals, which maintain that religion has negative effects on health–particularly for the vast majority of persons in the United States involved in mainstream Judeo-Christian beliefs and practices. Nevertheless, religion may be *used* by persons with mental disturbance or character pathology in negative and harmful ways. We have reviewed eight ways that religion can be abused in this manner. Because persons with mental illness may be more likely to use religion neurotically, it is not surprising that many mental health specialists conclude from their clinical observations that religion has negative effects on health. Such limited clinical observations, however, cannot be used to justify claims that religion causes health problems, nor can they be generalized to the vast majority of persons without mental illness in the United States who may use religious beliefs and practices adaptively to enhance both mental and physical health.

## REFERENCE NOTES

1. Koenig, H.G., L.K. George, and I. Siegler. (1988). The use of religion and other emotion-regulating coping strategies among older adults. *The Gerontologist* 28:303-310.

2. Koenig, H.G., H.J. Cohen, D.G. Blazer, C. Pieper, K.G. Meador, F. Shelp, V. Goli, R. DiPasquale. (1992). Religious coping and depression in elderly hospitalized medically ill men. *American Journal of Psychiatry* 149:1693-1700.

3. Koenig, H.G. (1996). Depressive disorder in hospitalized medically ill elders (unpublished data). Funded by National Institutes of Mental health, grant # MH01138 (1993-1998).

4. Manfredi, C., and M. Pickett. (1987). Perceived stressful situations and coping strategies utilized by the elderly. *Journal of Community Health Nursing* 4:99-110.

5. Rosen, C.E. (1982). Ethnic differences among impoverished rural elderly in use of religion as a coping mechanism. *Journal of Rural Community Psychology* 3:27-34.

6. Swanson, W.C., and C.L. Harter. (1971). How do elderly Blacks cope in New Orleans? *Aging and Human Development* 2:71-78.

7. Conway, K. (1985-1986). Coping with the stress of medical problems among black and white elderly. *International Journal of Aging and Human Development* 21:39-48.

8. Krause, N. (1995). Religiosity and self-esteem among older adults. *Journal of Gerontology* (Psychological Sciences) 50:P236-P246.

9. Pressman, P., J.S. Lyons, D.B. Larson, and J.S. Strain. (1990). Religious belief, depression, and ambulation status in elderly women with broken hips. *American Journal of Psychiatry* 147:758-760.

10. Nelson, P.B. (1989). Ethnic differences in intrinsic/extrinsic religious orientation and depression in the elderly. *Archives of Psychiatric Nursing* 3(4):199-204.

11. O'Connor, B.P., and R.J. Vallerand. (1990). Religious motivation in the elderly. A French-Canadian replication and an extension. *Journal of Social Psychology* 130:53-59.

12. Koenig, H.G. (1995). Religion and older men in prison. *International Journal of Geriatric Psychiatry* 10:219-230.

13. Koenig, H.G., J.N. Kvale, and C. Ferrel. (1988). Religion and well-being in later life. *The Gerontologist* 28:18-28.

14. Kivett, V.R. (1979). Religious motivation in middle age: Correlates and implications. *Journal of Gerontology* 34:106-115.

15. Wilson, M.R., and E.E. Filsinger. (1986). Religiosity and marital adjustment: multidimensional interrelationships. *Journal of Marriage and the Family* 48: 147-151.

16. Dudley, M.G., and F.A. Kosinski. (1990). Religiosity and marital satisfaction: A research note. *Review of Religious Research* 32:78-86.

17. Schumm, W.R., S.R. Bollman, and A.P. Jurich. (1982). The "marital conventionalization" argument: Implications for the study of religiosity and marital satisfaction. *Journal of Psychology and Theology* 10:236-241.

18. Robinson, L.C. (1994). Religious orientation in enduring marriage: an exploratory study. *Review of Religious Research* 35:207-218.

19. Sporakowski, M.J., and G.A. Hughston. (1978). Prescriptions for happy marriage: adjustments and satisfactions of couples married for 50 or more years. *The Family Coordinator* 321-327.

20. Roth, P.D. (1988). Spiritual well-being and marital adjustment. *Journal of Psychology and Theology* 16:153-158.

21. Rabins, P.V., M.D. Fitting, J. Eastham, and J. Zabora. (1990). Emotional adaptation over time in care-givers for chronically ill elderly people. *Age and Ageing* 19:185-190.

22. Koenig, H.G., J.C. Hays, L.K. George, and D.G. Blazer. (1996). Modeling the impact of chronic illness, religion, and social support on depressive symptoms. Paper presented at the *American Association for the Advancement of Science* annual meeting, Baltimore, Maryland, February 11, 1996.

23. Kennedy, G.J., H.R. Kelman, C. Thomas, and J. Chen. (1996). Religious affiliation, practice and depression among 1,855 older community residents. *Journal of Gerontology* (Psychological Sciences), in press.

24. Martin, W.T. (1984). Religiosity and United States suicide rates, 1972-1978. *Journal of Clinical Psychology* 40(5):1166-1169.

25. Stack, S. (1983). The effect of religiosity on suicide. *Journal for the Scientific Study of Religion* 22:239-252.

26. Koenig, H.G., S.M. Ford, L.K. George, D.G. Blazer, K.G. Meador. (1993). Religion and anxiety disorder: An examination and comparison of associations in young, middle-aged, and elderly adults. *Journal of Anxiety Disorders* 7:321-342.

27. Koenig, H.G., L.K. George, K.G. Meador, D.G. Blazer, and S.M. Ford. (1994). Religious practices and alcoholism in a southern adult population. *Hospital & Community Psychiatry* 45:225-237.

28. Beeghley, L., E.W. Bock, and J.K. Cochran. (1990). Religious change and alcohol use: An application of reference group and socialization theory. *Sociological Forum* 4:261-278.

29. Alexander, F., and R.W. Duff. (1991). Influence of religiosity and alcohol use on personal well-being. *Journal of Religious Gerontology* 8(2):11-21.

30. Miller, W.R. (1990). Spirituality: The silent dimension in addiction research. *Drug and Alcohol Review* 9:259-266.

31. Benson, P.L. (1992). Religion and substance use. In Schumaker, J.F. (Ed.) *Religion and Mental Health*. New York: Oxford University Press, pp. 211-220.

32. Ellison, C.G., and L.K. George. (1994). Religious involvement, social ties, and social support in a Southeastern community. *Journal for the Scientific Study of Religion* 33:46-61.

33. Ortega, S.T., R.D. Crutchfield, and W.A. Rushing. (1983). Race differences in elderly personal well-being. *Research on Aging* 5:101-118.

34. Blazer, D.G., and E. Palmore (1976). Religion and aging in a longitudinal panel. *Gerontologist* 16:82-85.

35. Krause, N., and T. Van Tran. (1989). Stress and religious involvement among older blacks. *Journal of Gerontology* 44:S4-13.

36. Ellison, C.G., D.A. Gay, and T.A. Glass. (1989). Does religious commitment contribute to individual life satisfaction. *Social Forces* 68:100-123.

37. Ellison, C.G. (1991). Religious involvement and subjective well-being. *Journal of Health and Social Behavior* 32:80-99.

38. Levin, J.S., L.M. Chatters, and R.J. Taylor. (1995). Religious effects on health status and life satisfaction among Black Americans. *Journal of Gerontology* (Social Sciences) 50B:S154-S163.

39. Guy, R.F. (1982). Religion, physical disabilities, and life satisfaction in older-age cohorts. *International Journal of Aging and Human Development* 15(3):225-232.

40. Usui, W.A.M., T.J. Keil, and K.R. Durig. (1985). Socioeconomic comparisons and life satisfaction of elderly adults. *Journal of Gerontology* 40:110-114.

41. Levin, J.S., K.S. Markides, and L.A. Ray. (1996). Religious attendance and psychological well-being in Mexican Americans: A panel analysis of three-generations data. *The Gerontologist*, in press.

42. Markides, K.S. (1983). Aging, religiosity, and adjustment: A longitudinal analysis. *Journal of Gerontology* 38:621-625.

43. Koenig, H.G. (1988). Religion and death anxiety in later life. *The Hospice Journal* 4(1):3-24.

44. Propst, L.R., R. Ostrom, P. Watkins, T. Dean, and D. Mashburn. (1992). Comparative efficacy of religious and nonreligious cognitive-behavioral therapy for the treatment of clinical depression in religious individuals. *Journal of Consulting and Clinical Psychology* 60:94-103.

45. Azhart, M.A., S.L. Varma, and A.S. Dharap. (1994). Religious psychotherapy in anxiety disorder patients. *Acta Psychiatrica Scandinavica* 90:1-3.

46. Idler, E.L. (1987). Religious involvement and the health of the elderly. *Social Forces* 66:226-238.

47. Idler, E.L., and S.V. Kasl. (1992). Religion, disability, depression, and the timing of death. *American Journal of Sociology* 97:1052-1079.

48. Yates, J.W., B.J. Chalmer, P. St. James, M. Follansbee, F.P. McKegney. (1981). Religion in patients with advanced cancer. *Medical and Pediatric Oncology* 9:121-128.

49. Van Reek, J., and M.J. Drop. (1986). Cigarette smoking in the U.S.A.: Sociocultural influences. *Rev Epidemiol Sante Publique* 34(3):168-173.

50. Larson, D.B., H.G. Koenig, B.H. Kaplan, R.S. Greenberg, E. Logue, and H.A. Tyroler. (1989). The impact of religion on men's blood pressure. *Journal of Religion and Health* 28:265-278.

51. Livingston, I.L., D.M. Levine, and R.D. Moore. (1991). Social integration and black intraracial variation in blood pressure. *Ethnicity and Disease* 1:135-149.

52. Graham, T.W., B.H. Kaplan, J.C. Cornoni-Huntley, S.A. James, C. Becker, C.G. Hames, and S. Heyden. (1978). Frequency of church attendance and blood pressure elevation. *Journal of Behavioral Medicine* 1(1):37-43.

53. Hutchinson, J. (1986). Association between stress and blood pressure variation in a Caribbean population. *American Journal of Physical Anthropology* 71:69-79.

54. Walsh, A. (1980). The prophylactic effect of religion on blood pressure levels among a sample of immigrants. *Social Sciences and Medicine* 14B:59-63.

55. Scotch, N.A. (1963). Sociocultural factors in the epidemiology of Zulu hypertension. *American Journal of Public Health* 53:1205-1213.

56. Armstrong, B., A. Merwyk, and H. Coates. (1977). Blood pressure in Seventh-Day Adventist vegetarians. *American Journal of Epidemiology* 105:444-449.

57. Colantonio, A., S.V. Kasl, and A.M. Ostfeld. (1992). Depressive symptoms and other psychosocial factors as predictors of stroke in the elderly. *American Journal of Epidemiology* 136:884-894.

58. Wardwell, W.I., C.B. Bahnson, and H.S. Caron. (1963). Social and psychological factors in coronary heart disease. *Journal of Health and Human Behavior* 4:154-165.

59. Comstock, G.W. (1971). Fatal arteriosclerotic heart disease, water hardness at home, and socioeconomic characteristics. *American Journal of Epidemiology* 94:1-10.

60. Comstock, G.W., and K.B. Partridge. (1972). Church attendance and health. *Journal of Chronic Disease* 25:665-672.

61. Medalie, J.H., H.A. Kahn, H.N. Neufeld, E. Riss, and U. Goldbourt. (1973). Five-year myocardial infarction incidence: II. Association of single variables to age and birthplace. *Journal of Chronic Disease* 26:329-349.

62. Phillips, R.L., F.R. Lemon, W.L. Beeson, and J.W. Kuzma. (1978). Coronary heart disease mortality among Seventh-Day Adventists with differing dietary habits: A preliminary report. *The American Journal of Clinical Nutrition* 31: S191-S198.

63. Lyon, J.L., H.P. Wetzler, J.W. Gardner, M.R. Klauber, and R.R. Williams. (1978). Cardiovascular mortality in Mormons and non-Mormons in Utah, 1969-1971. *American Journal of Epidemiology*, 108:5,357-366.

64. Friedlander, Y., J.D. Kark, and Y. Stein. (1986). Religious orthodoxy and myocardial infarction in Jerusalem: A case control study. *International Journal of Cardiology* 10:33-41.

65. Goldbourt, U., S. Yaari, and J.H. Medalie. (1993). Factors predictive of long-term coronary heart disease mortality among 10,059 male Israeli civil servants and municipal employees: A 23-year mortality followup in the Israeli Ischemic Heart Disease study. *Cardiology* 82:100-121.

66. Oxman, T.E., D.H. Freeman, and E.D. Manheimer. (1995). Lack of social participation or religious strength and comfort as risk factors for death after cardiac surgery in the elderly. *Psychosomatic Medicine* 57:5-15.

67. Zuckerman, D.M., S.V. Kasl, and A.M. Ostfeld. (1984). Psychosocial predictors of mortality among the elderly poor. The role of religion, well-being, and social contacts. *American Journal of Epidemiology* 119:410-423.

68. Byrd, R.C. (1988). Positive therapeutic effects of intercessory prayer in a coronary care unit population. *Southern Medical Journal* 81:826-829.

69. Enstrom, J.E. (1975). Cancer mortality among Mormons. *Cancer* 36:825-841.

70. Lyon, J.L., M.R. Klauber, J.W. Gardner, and C.R. Smart. (1976). Cancer incidence in Mormons and non-Mormons in Utah, 1966-1970. *New England Journal of Medicine* 294:129-133.

71. Jarvis, G.K. (1977). Mormon mortality rates in Canada. *Social Biology* 24:294-302.

72. Lyon, J.L., J.W. Gardner, M.R. Klauber, and C.R. Smart. (1977). Low cancer incidence and mortality in Utah. *Cancer* 39:2608-2618.

73. Enstrom, J.E. (1978). Cancer and total mortality among active Mormons. *Cancer* 42:1943-1951.

74. Dwyer, J.W., L.L. Clarke, and M.K. Miller. (1990). The effect of religious concentration and affiliation on county cancer mortality rates. *Journal of Health and Social Behavior* 31:185-202.

75. Phillips, R.L., J.W. Kuzma, W.L. Beeson, and T. Lotz. (1980). Influence of selection versus lifestyle on risk of fatal cancer and cardiovascular disease among Seventh-Day Adventists. *American Journal of Epidemiology* 112:296-314.

76. Phillips, R.L., and D.A. Snowden. (1983). Association of meat and coffee use with cancers of the large bowel, breast, and prostate among Seventh-Day Adventists: Preliminary results. *Cancer Research* 43(Supplement):2403s-2408s.

77. Berkel, J., and F. deWaard. (1983). Mortality pattern and life expectancy of Seventh-Day Adventists in the Netherlands. *International Journal of Epidemiology* 12:455-459.

78. Zollinger, T.W., R.L. Phillips, and J.W. Kuzma. (1984). Breast cancer survival rates among Seventh-Day Adventists and non-Seventh-Day Adventists. *American Journal of Epidemiology* 119:503-509.

79. Seidman, H. (1970). Cancer death rates by site and sex for religious and socioeconomic groups in New York City. *Environmental Research* 3:234-250.

80. MacMahon, B. (1960). The ethnic distribution of cancer mortality in New York City, 1955. *Acta-Unio Internationale Contra Cancrum* 16:1716-1724.

81. Herman, B., and P.E. Enterline. (1970). Lung cancer among the Jews and Non-Jews of Pittsburgh, Pennsylvania, 1953-1967: Mortality rates and cigarette smoking behavior. *American Journal of Epidemiology* 91:355-367.

82. Greenwald, P., R.F. Korns, P.C. Nasca, and P.E. Wolfgang. (1975). Cancer in United States Jews. *Cancer Research* 35:3507-3512.

83. Martin, A.O., J.K. Dunn, J.L. Simpson, C.L. Olsen, S. Kemel, M. Grace, S. Elias, G.E. Sarto, B. Smalley, and A.G. Steinberg. (1980). Cancer mortality in a human isolate. *Journal of the National Cancer Institute* 65:1109-1113.

84. Hamman, R.F., J.I. Barancik, and A.M. Lilienfeld. (1981). Patterns of mortality in the old order Amish: I. Background and major causes of death. *American Journal of Epidemiology* 114:845-861.

85. Larson, D.B., and H.G. Koenig. (1996). Does religion prolong your life? A systematic review of religion and mortality. *American Journal of Epidemiology*, in submission.

86. Pruyser, P. (1977). The seamy side of current religious beliefs. Bulletin of the Menninger Clinic 41:329-348.

87. Koenig, H.G., T. Lamar, and B. Lamar. (1997). *A Gospel for the Mature Years: Finding Fulfillment by Knowing and Using Your Gifts*. Binghamton, NY: The Haworth Press.

88. Andreasen, N.J.C. (1972). The role of religion in depression. *Journal of Religion and Health* 11:153-166.

# Chapter 8

# Implications

I have reviewed research that demonstrates a link between religion and health. The data strongly suggest, although they do not prove beyond all doubt, that the mature use of religion *causes* better health. What if we take one step beyond the data, however, and say that religion *is* good for health? Based on the research presented here, is this really such a bold leap? What if we say that a strong religious faith and active involvement in the religious community helps to prevent or reduce depression, anxiety, high blood pressure, stroke, heart attacks, cancer, and may add years to life? What might this mean for health professionals, clergy, public policymakers, medical researchers, and laypersons?

## *HEALTH PROFESSIONALS*

Demographic and societal trends in the remainder of this decade and early twenty-first century will greatly affect the way health care is provided. *Primary care physicians, nurses, and social workers* will be increasingly responsible for meeting the physical and mental health needs of a burgeoning population of middle-aged and older adults. This 74-million-member cohort of aging baby boomers may have high rates of physical health problems, depression, substance abuse, and other emotional disorders. By the year 2020, it is estimated that over 50 percent of all patients seen by physicians in this country will be over the age of 65. Because of the stigma associated with mental health problems, people are much more likely to seek mental health care from their personal physician than from a mental health specialist. Furthermore, managed care medicine, which is rapidly becoming the norm in this country, will require that all patients first see their primary care physician before seeking specialty care in the mental health sector (something that will be discouraged in order to limit health care costs).

As part of their role, health care providers are responsible for ensuring that the living situations of disabled, chronically ill patients are safe and that such persons receive adequate help performing basic self-care activities. With an increase in the number of persons with such needs in the years ahead, primary care physicians, nurses, and social workers–operating under increasing financial constraints–may become overwhelmed by the demand for such services. If families are unavailable, unable, or unwilling to help out, then health care providers may need to turn to other community organizations for assistance. Developing relationships and referral networks with religious congregations in the community may help ease the pressure on health care providers. Because of the importance of religion in the lives of so many Americans and its apparent positive effects on both physical and mental health, physicians, nurses, and social workers may be reassured that involving the religious community will seldom have ill effects and will likely enable them to provide better care for their patients.

Implications for *mental health professionals* are similar. Mental health specialists should question the teachings espoused by Freud, Ellis, Watters, and others, that devout religiousness, particularly that based in the Judeo-Christian tradition, leads to mental illness. These claims are based largely on anecdotal case reports, limited clinical experience, and largely personal bias. There is now almost overwhelming research evidence that religious belief and activity do not have negative effects on the mental health of most persons, but instead represent resources that may be turned to in order to help persons cope better with emotional distress. Some psychologists' and psychiatrists' negative experiences with religion in their clinical practices may result from the fact that persons with mental illness may be more likely to use religion in pathological ways (as described previously). Such neurotic uses of religion, however, cannot be generalized to the healthy use of religion, which the majority of Americans ascribe to. For this reason, mental health professionals should not be reluctant to develop relationships and referral networks with clergy in their community. In this way, each may assist and educate the other in sorting out healthy and pathological uses of religion.

What do the research findings mean for clinical practice? Health professionals might consider asking patients about their religious background, beliefs, and how these beliefs affect their health. This could be done as part of the initial patient encounter or comprehensive evaluation. Brief inquiries about religious issues could be made on subsequent visits to give patients permission to talk about any concerns they may have in this area. They will appreciate being allowed to discuss with their health providers religious concerns that may be vitally linked with health problems they are experiencing. Some patients may not feel comfortable talking with their minister about sensitive issues that have religious or moral connotations. Being supportive and respectful of patients' religious beliefs is essential at all times, even when they are at odds with the beliefs of the clinician or therapist. Health professionals must realize that these beliefs may be a tremendous source of strength to patients, which continues long after they leave the office. Consequently, they should encourage patients to actively participate in a faith community. This may reduce loneliness and isolation, and may reinforce religious beliefs that will help them to better cope with the stresses in their lives. Religious beliefs and practices may be integrated with or used adjunctively to traditional psychotherapy when treating patients with depression or anxiety disorders, and guidelines for such use of religion in therapy are being developed.[1,2]

Medical and psychiatric teams in acute care hospitals should include a chaplain as part of the health care team to ensure that religious and spiritual needs are met. The chaplain should be asked to provide meaningful input into medical, nursing, and social service care plans for each patient. Referral networks with clergy in the community will facilitate timely referral of members of the congregation with health problems early in the course of their disease, and also will enhance follow-up and compliance with treatment plans after patients are discharged back into the community.

## RELIGIOUS PROFESSIONALS

The days ahead will be as challenging for community pastors, chaplains, and pastoral counselors as it is for health care professionals. While there will be great opportunity to provide hope, encouragement, and direction to those struggling with health problems in their congregations and the wider community, this will also put a greater demand on their time and resources.

### Community Clergy

Pastors should be encouraged to present a contemporary message and style of worship that meets spiritual and psychological needs of persons with health and social problems. Members of the congregation should be directed and motivated to reach out to those in need both within and outside the church. As noted earlier, there will be increasing opportunity for pastors to work with health professionals to ensure that members of their congregations with mental or physical health problems are diagnosed promptly, treated appropriately, and followed up properly to ensure compliance and disease resolution. Increasing numbers of sick, disabled, vulnerable persons in the community who do not have supportive family, along with those who have fallen through the ever-widening cracks in our health care system, will come to the church for assistance. Pastors will need to be prepared to receive them and minister to their special needs.[3,4]

## *Chaplains*

Research demonstrating a strong relationship between religion and health should be particularly welcome to chaplains working in hospitals and other institutional settings. Because of the increasing pressure to limit costs, many chaplain positions are coming under increasing scrutiny by hospital administrators.[5] Chaplains are needing to justify their existence by showing that their services meet a need and help to reduce the cost of health care. Recent research is showing exactly that, with chaplain interventions reducing hospital stays,[6] decreasing recovery time after surgery,[7] cutting down on nursing time and increasing patient satisfaction,[8] and producing other financial savings for hospitals.[9,10] As noted earlier, chaplains should be included as active participants on health care teams, rounding with physicians and nurses and contributing to the development of health care plans.

Chaplains should also be active participants in nursing homes and other long-term care settings, which often have inconsistent relationships with community clergy. Not only should their tasks be to conduct religious services and pray with patients, but also it should be to provide counseling and support to those recently admitted or others who may be having difficulty adjusting to their new living situation. Such close contact with patients will provide an opportunity for chaplains to identify mental health problems that doctors and nurses might miss. To competently carry out their role, it is imperative that chaplains be knowledgeable about the diagnosis and treatment of mental disorders in middle-aged and older adults.[3,4]

### Pastoral Counselors

Well-designed research now shows that integrating religious beliefs and practices into psychotherapy for depressed or anxious religious patients actually produces faster results than secular techniques alone. This is validating for pastoral counselors and underscores the effectiveness of their methods. Religious faith, worship, prayer, and scripture reading are sometimes undervalued or even ridiculed by the "educated" public and many health professionals who are unaware of their value. Likewise, many pastoral counselors themselves have doubted the therapeutic value of traditional religious beliefs and practices, and have turned instead to modern secular techniques when counseling those who are suffering. If anything, the research in this book demonstrates the importance, value, and power that traditional religious beliefs and practices have on achieving and maintaining emotional and physical health. As with community clergy and chaplains, knowledge about the diagnosis and treatment of common mental and physical health problems in middle-aged and older adults is necessary for pastoral counselors to meet the special needs of this population.[3,4]

## PUBLIC POLICYMAKERS

Public policy experts should be particularly interested in the association between religion and health, given that before long, Medicare and other welfare programs will not be able to keep up with our health care needs–which by the year 2000 will cost the country nearly 2 trillion dollars, almost one-fifth of the entire economic output of the United States. Alternative health resources within our communities must be identified and alliances built in order to help take the pressure off government programs. Religious bodies can contribute in a number of ways to the health of communities. Already a number of joint ventures between local service agencies and churches have shown that this can be done and with good results.[11]

## *MEDICAL RESEARCHERS*

While much work has been done, much remains for the future. Important questions need answering. Each of the pathways in the model presented in Figure 6.2 need testing in order to refine our understanding of the mechanisms by which devout religious beliefs and practices affect health. How do religious belief and practice affect the use of general medical and mental health services? What religious beliefs and practices are most common among persons in good mental health? What religious beliefs and practices are most common among persons in good mental health despite having undergone major developmental traumas, adult life crises, or disabling physical illnesses? How can the healthy components of religion be integrated into psychotherapy with religious patients, and what aspects of religious belief and practice are most therapeutic in this regard?

More randomized clinical trials are needed to examine the effects of religious interventions (prayer, scripture reading, healing services) in persons with depression, anxiety, and other mental disorders. These studies are necessary to determine which types of religious intervention are most effective for which subgroups of patients. Likewise, studies are needed to determine how community mental health agencies, social services, and religious organizations might best work together. Pilot projects are needed to test collaborative ventures in order to identify and solve the inevitable problems that will arise. Finally, what is the best way to educate medical and psychiatric professionals about the contributions that clergy can make to patient care? Likewise, what is the best way to educate clergy about the services that mental health professionals provide and when to refer members of their congregations to them?

## *LAYPERSONS*

Becoming religious, only in order to gain positive effects on health, will probably not work very well. Research has shown that persons who use religion as a means to an end do not experience the psychological benefits of religious practice.[12,13] Rather, it is those who involve themselves in religion as an end in itself (i.e., persons with intrinsic faith) who are more likely to experience mental health, greater life satisfaction, and less worry and anxiety. For example, after examining the relationship between religious activities and death anxiety, Alvarado and colleagues concluded that "attempting to lower one's death anxiety or death depression by greater religious participation is not a guaranteed remedy . . . [Instead] perhaps faith, belief, and commitment must come before one experiences a lowering of death discomfort."[13] Thus, in order to achieve the health benefits I have been describing, persons may need to seek religion for religion's sake rather than for health reasons.

We are learning that middle-aged and older adults can best achieve and maintain emotional well-being if they use their talents and abilities to serve the needs of others in their church and larger community. As noted above, clergy are likely to be overwhelmed by demands on their time from increasing numbers of aging persons with mental and physical health needs in their congregations. Pastors will require the support and involvement of lay members of their churches in order to meet these needs. Research has shown that persons who provide support to others have higher well-being than those who do not.[14-16] "Loving thy neighbor as thyself" may indeed have health benefits. Nevertheless, there are numerous barriers and pitfalls that discourage people from reaching out and ministering to the needs of others around them, and burnout is a common phenomenon among such well-meaning caregivers. Strategies for overcoming these barriers and avoiding burnout, however, are being developed.[17]

## SUMMARY

In this chapter, I have discussed the implications of religion's effects on health for professionals and for laypersons. The research findings reviewed here have direct relevance on the day-to-day work of primary care physicians, nurses, social workers, psychiatrists, psychologists, counselors, pastors, chaplains, and pastoral counselors. While further research needs to be done, religious beliefs and practices may be a rich resource that persons can draw on to enhance both mental and physical health. The crisis in health care that looms ahead requires that we understand more about religion's effects on health. If further evidence continues to show that these effects are indeed positive, then we will need to actively encourage cooperation and collaboration between health care providers and the clergy.

## REFERENCE NOTES

1. Koenig, H.G., D.B. Larson, and D. Matthews. (1996). Religion and psychotherapy with older adults. *Journal of Geriatric Psychiatry* 29:155-184.

2. Propst, L.R. (1987). *Psychotherapy in a Religious Framework: Spirituality in the Emotional Healing Process.* NY: Human Sciences Press.

3. Koenig, H.G., and A.J. Weaver. (1997). *Counseling Troubled Older Adults: A Handbook for Pastors and Religious Caregivers.* Decator, GA: Abington Press (Academic Books).

4. Koenig, H.G., and A.J. Weaver. (1997). *Ministering to the Health Needs of Older Adults: What Pastors and Congregations Want to Know.* Minneapolis, MN: Augsburg-Fortress Press (in preparation).

5. Koenig, H.G. (1994). *Aging and God.* Binghamton, NY: The Haworth Press, pp. 303-304.

6. Florell, J.L. (1973). Crisis intervention in orthopedic surgery: empirical evidence of the effectiveness of chaplain working with surgery patients. *Bulletin of the American Protestant Hospital Association* 37:29.

7. McSherry, E., R. Fitzgerald, and H. Heffernan. (1995). Chaplains and the healthcare CEO. Paper presented at the NIH Conference on Spirituality and Health Care Outcomes, NIH, Bethesda, MD (March 22, 1995).

8. Parkum, K.H. (1985). The impact of chaplaincy services in selected hospitals in the eastern United States. *Journal of Pastoral Care* 39:262.

9.McSherry, E. (1987). The need and appropriateness of measurement and research in chaplaincy: Its criticalness for patient care and chaplain department survival post-1987. *Journal of Health Care Chaplaincy* 1:3-41.

10. Gartner, J.G., J.S. Lyons, D.B. Larson, J. Serkland, and M. Peyrot. (1990). Supplier-induced demand for pastoral care services in the general: A natural experiment. *Journal of Pastoral Care* 44(3):266-270.

11. Saunders, E. (1996). Church-based interventions for hypertension control. Paper presented at the Spiritual Intervention in Clinical Practice conference, sponsored by the National Institute for Healthcare Research at Landsdowne, Virginia (April 20, 1996).

12. Batson, C.D., and W.L. Ventis. (1982). *The Religious Experience.* New York: Oxford University Press.

13. Alvarado, K.A., D.I. Templer, C. Bresler, and S. Thomas-Dobson. (1995). The relationship of religious variables to death depression and death anxiety. *Journal of Clinical Psychology* 51:202-204.

14. Krause, N. (1987). Chronic financial strain, social support, and depressive symptoms among older adults. *Psychology and Aging* 2:185-192.

15. Krause, N., Herzog, A.R., and E. Baker. (1992). Providing support to others and well-being in later life. *Journal of Gerontology* 47:P300-P311.

16. Hays, J.C., L.R. Landerman, L.K. George, E.P. Flint, H.G. Koenig, D. Blazer, (1996). Social risk to mood states in late life. Based on data from Established Populations for Epidemiologic Studies in the Elderly (EPESE). Durham, NC: Duke University Medical Center.

17. Koenig, H.G., T. Lamar, and B. Lamar. (1997). *A Gospel for the Mature Years: Finding Fulfillment by Knowing and Using Your Gifts.* Binghamton, NY: The Haworth Press.

# General Reviews
# of the Research Literature

Bergin, A.E. (1983). Religiosity and mental health: A critical reevaluation and meta-analysis. *Professional Psychology: Research and Practice* 14:170-184.

Ellison, C.G., D.A. Gay, and T.A. Glass. (1989). Does religious commitment contribute to individual life satisfaction? *Social Forces* 68:100-123.

Futterman, A., and H.G. Koenig. (1995). Measuring religiosity in later life: What can gerontology learn from the sociology and psychology of religion? Background paper, published in proceedings of *Conference on Methodological Approaches to the Study of Religion, Aging, and Health*, sponsored by the National Institute on Aging (March).

Gartner, J., D. Larson, and G. Allen. (1991). Religious commitment and mental health: A review of the empirical literature. *Journal of Psychology and Theology* 19:6-25.

Koenig, H.G., M. Smiley, and J.P. Gonzales. (1988). *Religion, Health and Aging.* New York: Greenwood Press.

Koenig, H.G. (1995). *Research on Religion and Aging.* New York: Greenwood Press.

Koenig, H.G., and A. Futterman. (1995). Religion and health outcomes: A review and synthesis of the literature. Background paper, published in proceedings of *Conference on Methodological Approaches to the Study of Religion, Aging, and Health*, sponsored by the National Institute on Aging (March).

Larson, D.B., and S.S. Larson. (1994). *The Forgotten Factor in Physical and Mental Health: What Does the Research Show?* Rockville, MD: National Institute for Healthcare Research.

Levin, J.S., and P.L. Schiller. (1987). Is there a religious factor in health? *Journal of Religion and Health* 26:9-36.

Levin, J.S. (1995). Bibliography of gerontological research on religion. Supported by the Behavioral and Social Research program at the National Institute on Aging. Published in proceedings of *Conference on Methodological Approaches to the Study of Religion, Aging, and Health*, sponsored by the National Institute on Aging (March).

Matthews, D.A., and D.B. Larson. (1993-1996). *The Faith Factor: An Annotated Bibliography of Clinical Research on Spiritual Subjects.* Vols. I-IV. Rockville, MD: National Institute for Healthcare Research.

Schumaker, J.F. (1992). *Religion and Mental Health.* New York: Oxford University Press.

# Index

Page numbers followed by the letter "f" indicate a figure.

Activity (religious), 102
Affiliation (religious), 37-38,39f,40f
Agency (surrender of), 107
Aging parents, and geographic
    isolation, 16
Aging and religion, 44-46
    well-being in older adults, 54f
Aggression (rationalization for),
    105-106
Albert Einstein College of Medicine,
    59
Alcoholics Anonymous, 66,70
Alcoholism. *See also* Substance
    abuse
    and church attendance, 65f
    and lifetime disability, 15f
All-cause mortality, 92-93
Alvarado, K.A., 126
Alzheimer's disease, 12
    number of cases of, 12f
American Institute of Public
    Opinion, 45
*American Journal of Psychiatry*, 57
American Psychological
    Association, 28
Andreason, Nancy, 111
Anxiety, 63
    and church attendance, 64f
Applebaum, R.A., 11
Attendance (church), 38,40-43,41f
    and alcoholism, 65f
    and anxiety disorder, 64f
    and social support, 68
    and stroke, 86f
    and suicide rates, 62f

"Baby boomers," 10,14,18
Baker, Jim, 43
Balm of Gilead, *x*
Barna, George, 42
Belief (religious), 33-34,34f,35f,36
Mrs. Bernard (story), 2,5-7
Bible, 6,44
Blood vessels (disease of), 82-90
Body (displacement to), 108
Byrd, Randolph, 89

Cancer, 90-92
    death rates from by religious
        group, 91f
*Cardiology*, 87
Chaplains, 123-124
Character traits (reinforcement
    of undesirable), 109
Characteristics of religiosity, 26
Church
    attendance, 38,40-43,41f,102
        and alcoholism, 65f
        and anxiety disorder, 64f
        and social support, 68
        and stroke, 86f
        and suicide rates, 62f
    membership, 39
*Churches That Abuse*, 109
Clinical practice (implications for),
    121-122
Cognitive-behavioral psychotherapy
    (CBT), 67
Comfort, religion as a source of, 6
Commitment to religion, 102
Community clergy, 122-123

Community resources, 19
Comstock, George, 86
Control over self, loss of, 107
Coping, 6,55,56,102
    religious, 50-51,52f,53
        and severity of illness, 53f
Cornell, George, 41
Covalt, Nina, 28
Crisis of mental health, 13f
Cults (religious), 101

Deadly doctrine, *x*
*Deadly Doctrine*, 26,59,61
Demographic trends, 10
Dependency
    adult parents on children, 16
    promotion of excessive, 106-107
Depression, 13,55-60,61,63
    and Ellis, Albert, 25-26
    in hospitalized patients, 57f
    interventions for, 102
    predictions of change in, 58f
    and religion, 60f
*Diagnostic and Statistical Manual
    of Mental Disorders
    (DSM-III-R)*, 27
Direct mechanisms, 80
Direct religious influences, 78,80
    effects of, 80-81
Disability
    and alcoholism, 15
    and depression, 14f
    projected number of persons
        with, 11f
Disavowal (surrender of), 107
Discouragement of self-acceptance,
    26
Dissociation (surrender of), 107
Drug abuse. *See* Substance abuse
Duke University, 1,7,45,59
    Medical Center, 49,50
Dwyer, J.W., 91

Economic trends, 17-18
Effect, possible mechanisms
    of, 67-71
Effects of religion on health, 23-30
Egosyntonism, 109
Einstein, Albert, 1
Elderly
    federal funding of health care
        for, 18f
    parents geographically isolated
        from children, 16
Ellis, Albert, 2,33,49,111,120
    characteristics of religiosity, 26
    and depression, 25-26
Ellison, Christopher, 55
Enroth, Ronald, 109
Evans County (Georgia)
    Cardiovascular Study, 83
Excessive dependency (promotion
    of), 106-107

Faith, and health, 1
Faith healing, 29
Family trends, 15-17
Fanatical commitments (promotion
    of), 26
Fountain of Youth, *ix,xii*
*Free Inquiry*, 26
Freud, Sigmund, 2,23-25,33,46,49,
    71,110,111,120
Friedlander, Y., 87
Futterman, Andrew, 54
*Future of an Illusion*, 23

Generalizing across religious groups,
    70
Generation X, 18
Geographic isolation, 16
Geriatric Depression Scale, 56
*Geriatrics*, 28
God, belief in, 33-36,45
Goldbourt, U., 87
Government welfare programs, 17
Guilt, 68

Hamilton Depression Rating Scale, 56
Hatred (rationalization for), 105-106
Health
  Christianity and, *xi*
  and faith, 1
  and primary care physicians, 28-29
  and religion, *xi*
    direct effects of, 80-81
    negative effects of, 23-30
    and social trends, 9
Health care
  federal funding for the elderly, 18f
Health professionals, implications for, 119-122
Heart disease, 82-87,89-90
  mortality following cardiac surgery, 89f
  and religion, 88f
High blood pressure, 83-84
  and religiousness, 84f
Hoge Intrinsic Religiosity Scale, 53

Importance of religion, 36
Indirect mechanisms, 80
Indirect religious influences, 78,80
  effects of, 81-82
Influence (religion as)
  on health, *xii*
    negative, 23-30
    and social trends, 9
  on life, 36-37
Intellect, sacrifice for, 105
Interventions for depression, 102
Intolerance of others (promotion of), 26

Jones, Jim, 107
Jonestown massacre, 101
*Journal of Consulting and Clinical Psychology*, 25
Judgmental (justification for being), 107

Kaplan, H.G., 59
Kennedy, G.J., 59
Koenig, Harold G., *ix,x,xi,xii*
Koresh, David, 107
Kraus, N., 59,61
Kunkel, S.R., 11

*Lancet*, 29
Larson, David B., *ix*
Laypersons (implications for), 126-127
Levin, Jeffrey S., *ix,*55,59,61,77
Life, influence of religion on, 36-37
Life satisfaction, 53-55

Marital success, and religion, 69
Masochism, 108
"Me" generation, 16
Mechanisms of effect (possible), 67-71
Medalie, Jack, 86,87
Medicaid, 17
Medical researchers (implications for), 125-126
Medicare, 17
  Hospitalization Insurance Fund, 17
Membership (church), 38
Mental health. *See also* Depression
  and characteristics of religiosity, 26
  church attendance
    and anxiety disorder, 64f
    and suicide rates, 62f
  Ellis, Albert, 2,25-26
  Freud, Sigmund, 2,23-25
  future crisis, 13f
  and religion, *x,*49-50,101-102
    influences of, *xii*
    positive association, 60f
  Sarason, Seymour, 28
  Watters, Wendell, 2,26-27
Mental health professionals, implications for, 120-122

Morale, 53
Mortality
  all-cause, 92-93
  following cardiac surgery, 89f
  and religion, 78f

Narcissism, 109
National Institute on Aging, 54,58
National Institute of Mental Health
    (NIMH), 59,63,64
Negative effects of religion
  on health, 23-30
NIMH. *See* National Institute
  of Mental Health

Oates, Wayne, 109
Obsessional thinking, 108-109
Oxman, Thomas, 87

Parents
  geographic isolation
    from children, 16
Pastoral counselors, 124
Pathological aspects of religion,
    104-105,109
Philadelphia Geriatric Morale Scale,
    53
Phillips, R.L., 87
Physical health
  and religion, *x*,77-78,102-104
    influences of, *xii*
      direct effects of, 80-81
      indirect effects of, 81-82
      prevention model for, 79f
Prayer, *xi*,43-44
Predictors of well-being, 61
Prejudice (rationalization for),
    105-106
Prevention model for religion's
    influence on physical health,
    79f
Primary care physicians, 28-29

Princeton Religion Research Center
    Index, 40
Promotion of excessive dependency,
    106-107
Pruyser, Paul, 104,108
*Psychosomatic Medicine*, 87
*Psychosomatics*, 57
Public Policymakers, 124-125

Reinforcement of undesirable
    character traits, 109
Reliance on God (encouragement
    of), 26
Religion. *See also* Prayer
  and aging, 44-46
  church
    attendance, 38,40-43,41f
    membership, 38
  commitment to, 102
  and coping, 50-51,52f,53
    and severity of illness, 53f
  and the fountain of youth, *xiii*
  importance of, 36
  influence on health, *xii*
    direct/indirect, 78,80
      effects of, 80-81,82
    negative, 23-30
    prevention model for, 79f
    and social trends, 9
  influence on life, 36-37
  and marital success, 69
  and mental health,
      *x*,49-50,101-102
    positive association, 60f
    severity of mental illness, 53f
  and mortality, 78f
  neurotic, 23
  pathological aspects of, 26,
      104-105,109
  and physical health, *x*,77-78,
      102-104
  as a source of comfort, 6
  and sports, 41-42
  and substance abuse, 66
  and television, 43

Religion *(continued)*
  and well-being in older adults, 54f
Religiosity, characteristics of, 26
Religious activity, 102
Religious affiliation, 37-38,39f,40f
Religious beliefs, 33-34,34f,35f,36
Religious CBT, 67
Religious Coping Index, 56
Religious cults, 101
*Religious Factors in Mental Illness*,
  109
Religious groups, generalizing
  across, 70
Religious professionals, implications
  for, 122-124
Religiousness and high blood
  pressure, 84f
Research implications
  and health professionals, 119-122
  and laypersons, 126-127
  and medical researchers, 125-126
  and public policymakers, 124-125
  and religious professionals,
    122-124
Risk-taking (discouragement of), 26

Sacrifice for intellect, 105
Sarason, Seymour, 28
Scientific method, to study mental
  health and religiousness,
  49-50
Secular CBT, 67
Self-esteem, 61
Self-rated scale, 53
Social security, 17
Social support, 69
  and church attendance, 68
Social trends
  community resources, 19
  demographic, 10

Social trends *(continued)*
  economic, 17-18
  family, 15-17
  health, 11-15
    and religious influences on, 9
Spiegel, David, 81
Spirituality, 70-71
Sports and religion, 41-42
Standard depression scales, 56
Standard treatment protocol, 67
Stroke, 84-85
  and church attendance, 86f
Substance abuse, 63-66
  church attendance and alcoholism,
    65f
Suicide. *See also* Depression
  and church attendance, 62f

Television (religious), 43
*Textbook of Psychiatry*, 59
Thought control, 106-107
Treatment studies, 66-67,80

Undesirable character traits
  (reinforcement of), 109

Vaillant, George, 66

Waco disaster, 101
Wardwell, W.I., 86
Watters, Wendell, 2,26-27,33,49,59,
  61,111,120
Well-being, 53-55
  predictors of, 61
  and religion in older adults, 54f

Zuckerman, D.M., 93

# Order Your Own Copy of
## This Important Book for Your Personal Library!

---

## IS RELIGION GOOD FOR YOUR HEALTH?
### The Effects of Religion on Physical and Mental Health

_____ in hardbound at $39.95 (ISBN: 0-7890-0166-7)

_____ in softbound at $19.95 (ISBN: 0-7890-0229-9)

---

COST OF BOOKS_____

OUTSIDE USA/CANADA/
MEXICO: ADD 20%_____

POSTAGE & HANDLING_____
*(US: $3.00 for first book & $1.25
for each additional book)*
*Outside US: $4.75 for first book
& $1.75 for each additional book)*

SUBTOTAL_____

IN CANADA: ADD 7% GST_____

STATE TAX_____
*(NY, OH & MN residents, please
add appropriate local sales tax)*

**FINAL TOTAL**_____
*(If paying in Canadian funds,
convert using the current
exchange rate. UNESCO
coupons welcome.)*

☐ **BILL ME LATER:** ($5 service charge will be added)
(Bill-me option is good on US/Canada/Mexico orders only;
not good to jobbers, wholesalers, or subscription agencies.)

☐ Check here if billing address is different from
shipping address and attach purchase order and
billing address information.

Signature_____

☐ **PAYMENT ENCLOSED: $**_____

☐ **PLEASE CHARGE TO MY CREDIT CARD.**

☐ Visa   ☐ MasterCard   ☐ AmEx   ☐ Discover
☐ Diner's Club

Account #_____

Exp. Date_____

Signature_____

Prices in US dollars and subject to change without notice.

NAME_____

INSTITUTION_____

ADDRESS_____

CITY_____

STATE/ZIP_____

COUNTRY_____ COUNTY (NY residents only)_____

TEL_____ FAX_____

E-MAIL_____

May we use your e-mail address for confirmations and other types of information? ☐ Yes   ☐ No

*Order From Your Local Bookstore or Directly From*
**The Haworth Press, Inc.**
10 Alice Street, Binghamton, New York 13904-1580 • USA
TELEPHONE: 1-800-HAWORTH (1-800-429-6784) / Outside US/Canada: (607) 722-5857
FAX: 1-800-895-0582 / Outside US/Canada: (607) 772-6362
E-mail: getinfo@haworth.com
PLEASE PHOTOCOPY THIS FORM FOR YOUR PERSONAL USE.

BOF96